CANDID: Camberwell Ass of Need for Adults with Developmental and Intellectual Disabilities

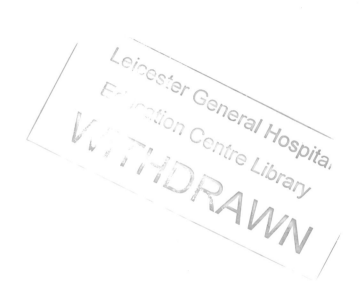

CANDID: Camberwell Assessment of Need for Adults with Developmental and Intellectual Disabilities

A needs assessment for people with learning disabilities and mental health problems

Kiriakos Xenitidis
Mike Slade
Graham Thornicroft
Nick Bouras

Published by Gaskell
London

Gaskell is an imprint of the Royal College of Psychiatrists,
17 Belgrave Square, London SW1X 8PG

Gaskell is a registered trademark of the Royal College of Psychiatrists.

British Library Cataloguing-in-Publication Data
A catalogue record for this book is available from the British Library.

ISBN 1-901242-99-4

Distributed in North America by Balogh International, Inc.

The views presented in this book do not necessarily reflect those of the Royal College of Psychiatrists, and the publishers are not responsible for any error of omission or fact.

The Royal College of Psychiatrists is a registered charity (no. 228636)

Printed in the UK by Cromwell Press Ltd, Trowbridge, Wiltshire.

Contents

Acknowledgements

Interviews to evaluate the CANDID were undertaken by Helen Philp, Jane Sayer, Elizabeth Harris and Donna McGee. Maria Fotiadou and Declan Murphy contributed at various stages in the development of the CANDID. The invaluable statistical advice from Morven Leese is acknowledged.

The authors are grateful to Karen Langridge (at PRiSM) and Chris Laming (at ESTIA) who provided expert administrative support.

The authors would like to thank all the service users, carers and staff members who took part in the validity and reliability study. Without their contribution, the CANDID development project would not have been possible.

Contributors

Kiriakos Xenitidis — Consultant Psychiatrist & Honorary Senior Lecturer, South London & Maudsley NHS Trust and Institute of Psychiatry

Mike Slade — MRC Clinician Scientist Fellow, Section of Community Psychiatry (PRiSM), Health Services Research Department, Institute of Psychiatry

Graham Thornicroft — Professor of Community Psychiatry, Section of Community Psychiatry (PRiSM), and Head of Health Services Research Department, Institute of Psychiatry

Nick Bouras — Professor of Psychiatry and Honorary Consultant Psychiatrist, Guy's King's & Thomas' School of Medicine / Institute of Psychiatry and South London & Maudsley NHS Trust

List of abbreviations

CAN   Camberwell Assessment of Need
CANDID   Camberwell Assessment of Need for Adults with Developmental and Intellectual Disabilities
CANDID–R   CANDID – Research Version
CANDID–S   CANDID – Short Version
CANE   Camberwell Assessment of Need for the Elderly
CANFOR   Camberwell Assessment of Need – Forensic Version (including CANFOR–S, CANFOR–C and CANFOR–R)
PRiSM   The Psychiatric Research in Service Measurement team is the Section of Community Psychiatry at the Institute of Psychiatry, London
ESTIA   The Evaluation, Support, Training, Intervention and Assessment Team is the academic component of the Mental Health in Learning Disabilities department at Guy's Hospital

1 Introduction

The *Camberwell Assessment of Need for Adults with Developmental and Intellectual Disabilities* (CANDID) is a needs assessment scale specifically designed for people with learning disabilities (mental retardation, mental handicap or mental impairment) and mental health problems. The CANDID was developed at the Institute of Psychiatry, London, by modification of the *Camberwell Assessment of Need* (CAN), an established needs assessment scale for people with severe and enduring mental illness (Slade *et al*, 1999). The validity and reliability of the CAN and CANDID have been investigated by Phelan *et al* (1995) and Xenitidis *et al* (2000), respectively and were found to be acceptable. Two further variants of the CAN have been developed: one for use with older adults (CANE; Orrell & Hancock, 2004) and a forensic CAN (CANFOR; Thomas *et al*, 2003).

Two versions of the CANDID have been developed: a research version (CANDID–R) and a short version (CANDID–S), for both research and clinical use. The CANDID, in both its versions, is a screening instrument that aims to identify areas of need, which may then be explored further by the appropriate person or team using more detailed instruments as necessary. If, for example, an unmet Mobility need is identified, a full assessment by a physiotherapist may be required. Both versions of the CANDID are administered by a semi-structured interview enquiring about need in 25 life domains. A time frame of 4 weeks prior to the interview is used. The CANDID–S is a brief (one page) schedule that aims to establish for each domain: i) whether a need is present; and ii) where a need exists, whether it is currently met or unmet. The CANDID–R addresses in addition the issues of help received for each need from both professional and informal carers, how much help is needed and whether the respondent is satisfied with the help the person is currently receiving.

The CANDID covers a wide range of physical and mental health needs as well as social needs. It records the views of the service users and their carers in addition to those of staff. The CANDID can be used by (i) people who are involved in the care of adults with learning disabilities (either professionally or informally); and (ii) people interested in evaluating learning disabilities services (e.g. researchers, managers).

This book provides a brief introduction to the subject of needs assessment in learning disabilities services (Chapter 2), a description of the process of development of the CANDID (Chapter 3), detailed instructions for using the two versions of the instrument (Chapters 4 & 5) and help with rating either version (Chapter 7). Chapter 6 contains guidance for training interviewers in the use of the CANDID. The full instruments can be found in Appendices 1 and 2, which can be photocopied for clinical or research use. Also included for photocopying are the rating sheets for CANDID–R (Appendix 3) and material to facilitate training in the use of CANDID (Appendices 4 & 5). Finally, the paper published in the *British Journal of Psychiatry* reporting on the validity and reliability of the CANDID is included in Appendix 6.

Chapters 4 and 5 are intended to be self-contained, so the duplication between the two chapters and a degree of overlap with other chapters is intentional. Those wishing to use the CANDID for *clinical* purposes are advised to read Chapters 2 and 3 for background and then use the CANDID–S (Appendix 1) according to the instructions contained in Chapter 4. However, the CANDID–R (Appendix 2) contains a wider range of prompting questions and can be used for the CANDID–S interviewers to familiarise themselves with the interviewing style and questions. Those intending to use the CANDID in a *research* project may choose to use the CANDID–S or CANDID–R, depending on whether the additional information elicited by the CANDID–R is required for the particular research study. Instructions for the use of CANDID–R can be found in Chapter 5.

2 Needs assessment in learning disabilities mental health services

Definitions and policy background

The increased risk that people with learning disabilities will develop mental health problems compared to the general population has only in recent years become the focus of interest among mental health professionals. There was a widely held belief that people with learning disabilities were not capable of developing mental illness like the rest of the population. Moreover, the behavioural disorders frequently exhibited by people with learning disabilities were attributed entirely to their impaired cognitive development (White *et al*, 1995). However, in the past two decades, consensus has emerged that learning disabilities and mental illness can co-exist, and that people with learning disabilities are more susceptible than the general population to developing a wide range of mental health problems (Eaton & Menolascino, 1982; Sovner & Hurley, 1983; Reiss, 1994).

The National Health Service & Community Care Act 1990 in the UK distinguished between 'social care' and 'health care' and charged social services with the obligation to conduct a needs assessment of any individual who may require community care. Although there seems to be agreement about the importance of providing services according to need, there is a lack of consensus about the *definition of need*. Among the most relevant definitions of need for people with learning disabilities are 'the requirement of individuals to enable them to achieve acceptable quality of life' (Department of Health Social Services Inspectorate, 1991) and 'a problem which can benefit from an existing intervention' (Stevens & Gabbay, 1991). People with learning disabilities often have a complex constellation of difficulties, commonly referred to as 'special needs'. It has not, however, been established whether either of the previous definitions of need (or indeed any other) contain the necessary and sufficient information for defining need in this population. In addition, there is a lack of agreement as to *who should assess need*. Mooney (1986) suggests, from a health economics point of view, that need can be assessed only by professionals, whereas others (Bradshaw, 1972) use a sociological perspective to argue that individuals' assessment of their own needs are valid as 'felt' and 'expressed' needs. Slade (1994) highlighted, in the context of mental health services, the importance of taking the users' views into account, especially if they differ significantly from those of their carers or the professionals.

The planning and provision of mental health services for people with learning disabilities has been the subject of considerable discussion and change in recent years. The resettlement of adults with learning disabilities from large institutions to smaller residences in the community was accelerated in the UK as a result of recent legislation. These changes raise important issues relating to the delivery of services (Bouras & Holt, 2001), and have resulted in the case for the development of specialised mental health services for people with learning disabilities being advocated (Bouras, 1999; Hassiotis *et al*, 2000). The development of specialist teams has also been recommended by the Royal College of Psychiatrists (1996). Despite this, two recent national surveys in the UK revealed widespread deficits in local service planning and a variety of unmet mental health needs for people with learning disabilities (Gravestock & Bouras, 1997; Bailey & Cooper, 1998).

Recent UK government documents have acknowledged these limitations in care, and emphasised the need for modernising both the National Health Service as a whole (Department of Health, 1997) and mental health services in particular (Department of Health, 1999a). They highlighted the importance of planning and delivering 'safe, sound and supportive' services, by ensuring that service users are provided with the care they need at the time they need it. Thus, the importance of assessing individual needs has been emphasised. Needs assessment at the population level is also addressed in these policy initiatives and is described as 'an essential first step in planning services' (Department of Health, 1997). Apart from the importance of needs assessment at an individual and population level, the significance of undertaking this assessment in partnership between Local Authorities and Health Authorities is underlined, as people with learning disabilities and mental health problems often have complex needs that cross traditional organisational boundaries. Also, more recently mental health and learning disabilities services are increasingly commissioned jointly by Local and Health Authorities.

The Department of Health also published the National Service Framework for Mental Health (NSF–MH) (Department of Health, 1999b), a long-term strategic blueprint for services for adults with mental health problems for the next decade. The aims were to help drive up quality, remove the wide and unacceptable variations in provision, set national standards and define service models, put in place programmes to support local delivery, and establish milestones and performance indicators to measure progress (Thornicroft, 2000). Although specialist learning disability mental health services are not specifically referred to the principles, they are directly applicable to this population. The *National Strategy for Learning Disability Services* was published subsequently and sought to clarify issues and to complement the National Service Framework for Mental Health in the area of learning disability services (Department of Health, 2001).

Existing assessment instruments

A number of instruments have been developed to measure mental health problems and/or needs in people with learning disabilities. These instruments can be broadly divided into the following two categories:

Assessment tools for behavioural and mental health problems

The most commonly used instruments include:

a   *The Aberrant Behaviour Checklist (ABC)* (Aman et al, 1985), a research-oriented checklist of behavioural problems, originally developed for use as a treatment outcome measure.

b   *The Adaptive Behaviour Scale (ABS)* (Nihira et al, 1974), which was developed to be used for individual programme planning and evaluation of services. It is divided in two parts: Part I assesses adaptive functioning in 10 life domains and Part II assesses 14 types of maladaptive behaviour.

c   *The Reiss Screen for Maladaptive Behaviour* (Reiss, 1988), a screening instrument for behavioural problems.

d   *The Psychopathology Instrument for Mentally Retarded Adults (PIMRA)* (Kazdin et al, 1983), which focuses on psychiatric symptoms, and is available in self-report and informant versions.

e   *The Psychiatric Assessment Schedule for Adults with Developmental Disabilities (PAS–ADD)* (Moss et al, 1998), a psychopathology measure available in three versions.

Instruments for the assessment of needs for services

The following are commonly used instruments:

a   *The Hampshire Assessment for Living with Others (HALO)* (Shackleton-Bailey & Pidcock, 1983), which was developed to inform planning for residential placement and the training needs of people with learning disabilities.

b   *The Vineland Social Maturity Scale* (Doll, 1965), which was designed to assist the development of individual care programmes for children and adults with learning disabilities.

c   *The Disability Assessment Schedule (DAS)* (Holmes *et al*, 1982), a rating scale completed through interview with an informant that assesses impairments, skills and behaviour in 12 life domains.

d   *The Social Training Achievement Record (STAR)* (Williams, 1982), a measure of adaptive behaviour with acceptable validity and reliability, which was designed specifically for assessment prior to skills training.

e   *The Index of Social Competence* (McConkey & Walsh, 1982), which was designed for the needs of a specific research project.

f   *Pathways to Independence* (Jeffree & Cheseldine, 1982), a series of checklists of self-help, personal and social skills, designed to assess in detail skills in 11 life domains, with a focus on those needed for personal and social independence.

Inevitably, there is an overlap between the two categories as mental health or behavioural problems interfere with a variety of skills and generate needs for services. Thus, some primarily diagnostic or screening tools may indirectly assess needs for services. The above list is not meant to be a comprehensive review of existing measures. O'Brien *et al* (2001) reviewed the use of a number of assessment schedules. However, the majority of these instruments are lengthy, typically require special training for their administration and are completed by professionals only, so they do not take into consideration the views of service users or their carers. None of the above instruments has been designed specifically with the statutory requirement of needs assessment in mind (House of Commons, 1990).

The CANDID was developed to address the above issues and to meet the obligation on services to assess the needs of people with learning disabilities and mental health problems.

3 Development of the Camberwell Assessment of Need for Adults with Developmental and Intellectual Disabilities (CANDID)

Background and structure of the instrument

The CANDID was developed by modifying the *Camberwell Assessment of Need (CAN)* (Phelan *et al*, 1995; Slade *et al*, 1999) to specifically address the needs of adults with learning disabilities and mental health problems.

The four principles underlying the development of CANDID are that:

1   people with learning disabilities and mental health problems have basic needs like everybody else along with specific needs associated with their conditions
2   the primary aim is to identify rather than describe in detail each need; once a need is identified, more specialist assessment can be conducted in those domains
3   needs assessment should be possible to be conducted by a wide range of people, so that it can be applied in routine clinical practice
4   there may be differences of opinion about the existence of need among people involved and therefore different points of view should be recorded separately.

The criteria established during the process of the development of the CANDID were that it:

1   has known and acceptable validity and reliability
2   is brief and suitable for use by a range of professionals
3   requires no formal training
4   records the points of view of the service user, informal carer and staff
5   measures met and unmet need
6   measures the help provided by informal carers and services separately
7   is suitable for use in research and clinical practice using two separate versions.

Both versions of the CANDID are administered by a semi-structured interview enquiring about need in 25 life domains:

1   Accommodation
2   Food
3   Looking after the home
4   Self-care
5   Daytime activities
6   General physical health
7   Eyesight/hearing
8   Mobility
9   Seizures
10   Major mental health problems
11   Other mental health problems
12   Information
13   Exploitation risk
14   Safety of self
15   Safety of others
16   Inappropriate behaviour
17   Substance misuse
18   Communication
19   Social relationships
20   Sexual expression
21   Caring for someone else
22   Basic education
23   Transport
24   Money budgeting
25   Welfare benefits.

Assessment of each of the domains in the CANDID–R uses the same format of four sections.

Section 1   assesses the absence or presence of need, and if need is present, whether it is met or unmet.
Section 2   rates the help received from informal carers.
Section 3   assesses the respondent's views on:
    a   how much help local services are *providing*
    b   how much help the person *needs* from local services
Section 4   assesses the respondent's satisfaction with:
    a   the *type* of help received from local services
    b   (for non-staff respondents) the *amount* of help received from local services.

The CANDID–S is a brief (one-page) schedule that aims to establish for each domain first, whether a need is present and second, where a need exists, whether it is currently met or unmet. Thus, the CANDID–S only uses Section 1 with identical need ratings to the CANDID–R.

Psychometric properties

A research study investigating the reliability and validity of the CANDID has been conducted (Xenitidis *et al*, 2000) and the corresponding paper is reprinted in Appendix 6. Briefly, for testing the validity of the new instrument the views of the service users, their informal carers and professional experts were sought through a process of focus groups and surveys. The reliability of the CANDID was investigated both for the instrument as a whole (global reliability) and by an item-per-item comparison. To assess global reliability, intraclass correlations between summary scores of the two raters (for inter-rater reliability) and at two points in time (for test–retest reliability) were calculated using variance components analysis. For interrater reliability, the overall intraclass correlation coefficient (r) for the total number of needs was 0.93 for user ratings, 0.90 for carer ratings and 0.97 for staff ratings. For test–retest reliability the correlation coefficients were 0.71, 0.69 and 0.86, respectively. For item-per-item reliability (interrater and test–retest), the percentage range of complete agreement was between 71% and 100% and was generally higher for staff ratings and for interrater reliability. As described in the paper, the estimation of interrater reliability was based on two raters rating the same interview, as obtaining ratings of separate interviews was not possible due to methodological constraints.

The mean number of needs per service user identified by the member of staff was approximately 14 (out of maximum possible of 25). This was almost identical with that identified by the informal carer, and both were higher than the user's assessment of their own needs (11.5). The ratings of carers and staff did not differ significantly, whereas the differences between the ratings of users and carers as well as between users and staff were significant ($p < 0.01$).

The CANDID is brief and easy to administer by assessors from different professional backgrounds, and it does not require formal training for its administration. It measures met and unmet needs, and records the contribution of formal services and informal carers in meeting needs. It assesses the views of the service users themselves, their informal carers and members of staff involved in their care.

The findings of the CANDID validity and reliability study suggest that this instrument has acceptable validity and reliability when used under research conditions. More data are required on its utility and feasibility, which will be established with its longer-term application in routine settings.

4 Using the CANDID–S

What can CANDID–S be used for?

The CANDID–S (Appendix 1) is a short tool for the assessment of needs of people with learning disabilities and mental health problems. It can be used for clinical and research purposes. It identifies needs (met and unmet) in 25 domains of life, as described in Chapter 3.

The CANDID–S can be used for clinical purposes, in the development of individualised care plans in community and hospital settings. For example, a community team could use the CANDID–S routinely in initial assessments of new service users, to identify the range of domains in which they are likely to require further assessment and possibly help or treatment. Aggregated results from individual needs assessments can also be used to estimate the need of a defined population. CANDID–S data can be used for audit and service development purposes, such as investigating whether enough users have unmet needs in a particular domain (e.g. *Welfare benefits*) to make it worthwhile to employ relevant professionals (e.g. a welfare benefits advisor).

For research purposes, the CANDID–S can be used in studies for which the additional information provided in CANDID–R (Chapter 5) is not relevant or necessary. For example, CANDID–S can be used as a measure for investigating whether and why staff and service users' or carers' perceptions differ, or comparing the impact on needs of two different types of services.

Who can use CANDID–S?

Any person with experience in working with adults with learning disabilities and mental health problems can use CANDID–S. It can be completed by people from a variety of professional backgrounds including direct care workers, mental health professionals, social services practitioners, learning disabilities service planners, clinicians and researchers, etc. Although the interviewer needs to have experience of clinical assessment interviews and previous experience of using assessment schedules is helpful, formal training is not a requirement for using CANDID–S. The interviewer should become familiar with the entire questionnaire before the first use. Subsequent assessments as well as interrater reliability are expected to improve by perusing this chapter. This book can be used as the basis for in-house training (Chapter 6) if, taking into account the local circumstances, this is thought to be useful, prior to introducing CANDID–S in routine clinical practice or as a tool in a research project.

Whose views are assessed?

Three different perspectives can be assessed: those of the service *user* (patient, client, the person being assessed), informal *carer* (relative or friend) and *staff*. If an interview with the *user* is impossible, an advocate can be interviewed and instructed to answer the questions as if they were the user, rather than giving their own views. The informal *carer* can be anyone who is not paid for the care they provide, such as a relative or friend. The *staff* assessor could be any member of staff who has a good knowledge of the person's circumstances, such as a direct care worker, a day centre staff member, a community nurse, a psychiatrist, etc.

For clinical purposes, the user and carer columns are completed by the staff through interviewing the relevant person, and the staff member can separately complete the staff column with their own assessment or (if not directly involved in the person's care) through interviewing another relevant staff member. For research purposes, a researcher interviews the user and informal carer, and either interviews the staff or gives a copy to the staff (if familiar with the CANDID schedules) for self-completion. The assessments of user, carer and staff views can be in any order. Any of the three or all three assessments may be made.

With the exception of an advocate responding on behalf of the person being assessed, respondents should be encouraged to give their own views on the needs of the user. It is this view (not the view of the interviewer) that is recorded. The perspectives of users, carers and staff may differ – this is why their assessments are recorded in different columns.

How is CANDID–S used?

The interview/assessment with each respondent uses one column. The assessment procedure in each domain is identical. The suggested questions, shown in italics, may be used to open discussion in each of the 25 domains. Additional questions should be asked with the goal of establishing whether the user has a need (currently met or unmet) in this domain. The time frame used is the **4 weeks** prior to the interview.

Some of the opening questions that appear in the CANDID–R have been omitted from the CANDID–S in order to keep the instrument short. It is therefore recommended that interviewers familiarise themselves with the full Section 1 for each domain (shown in the CANDID–R). Inexperienced CANDID–S interviewers may find it helpful for the first few assessments to conduct the interview using Section 1 of the CANDID–R, while recording their ratings on the CANDID–S sheet.

To avoid confusion and repetition, each domain should be explored fully before questions about the next one are asked. However, it is not essential that the order of domains is followed rigidly. Thus, if the respondent or the interviewer finds that, for example, *Inappropriate behaviour* follows naturally from *Safety of self*, asking questions in this order may be preferred. It is, of course, important that questions on all 25 domains are asked.

Each interview typically takes approximately 10–15 minutes to administer. This time becomes shorter as the interviewer becomes more familiar with using the scale. The duration of the interview, however, may vary, depending on the number of identified needs of the person being assessed and the respondent's attributes (e.g. interviewing an anxious parent or a distractible service user may prolong the duration of the interview). An explanation should be given prior to commencing the interview that its purpose is to identify rather than describe in detail each area of need.

Rating guidelines

The definitions of met and unmet need in CANDID are based on the same principles as those adopted by the CAN (Slade *et al*, 1999).

A need is defined as met (need rating 1) when help is given for a particular problem and as a result of this, in the respondent's view:

a   the problem does not exist any more, OR

b   the problem is still present but only to a moderate degree, i.e. it does not constitute a serious problem any more.

A need in a particular domain is defined as unmet (need rating 2) if in the respondent's view:

a   there is a serious problem in this domain and no help is currently being given, OR

b   despite help there is still a serious problem.

Thus, for each **need rating,** there are four options based on the respondent's answers to the questions.

0=no need	no serious problem in this area & no help given
1=met need	no problem or only moderate problem due to help given
2=unmet need	serious problem exists, whether or not help is given
9=not known	the respondent does not know the answer or does not want to answer.

If the problem persists despite any help that the person is receiving in this domain, then the distinction between met need and unmet need is a matter of judgement regarding the severity of the problem. The goal is to differentiate between problems that are current and serious, and those that are of moderate severity and are ameliorated by help. However, there may still be a blurred boundary where the user is receiving help, which only partly addresses their difficulties. It is the respondent's assessment of the degree of the problem that will guide the rating. A good question to identify the respondent's assessment is 'On balance, would you say that in this area there is a *serious problem?*' If the problem is only moderate or under control with the help the user is getting, then the need rating is 1 (met need). If the problem is still considered to be current and severe, then the need rating is 2 (unmet need) (Chapter 7, question 7). An algorithm for making a need rating is also given in Chapter 7.

A response of 'no problem' requires further prompting to identify whether no problem exists because of help given (i.e. need rating 1 – met need), or no problem exists and no help is given (i.e. need rating 0 – no need). A rating of 1 is given if the reason for there being no problem is that the person is receiving help (i.e. there would be a problem if the help were to be withdrawn). A rating of 0 is given if the person is not receiving any help and still has no problem in this particular domain. A rating of 0 is also given if this domain does not apply to the user (see Chapter 7, question 1).

The CANDID–S makes no assumption that the reason for the existence of a need is the person's learning disability or mental health problems. Thus, if a person has not been able to use public transport in the past 4 weeks because of a physical illness, then the existence of a need in the Transport domain should be recorded and a rating of 1 or 2 should be given (see Chapter 7, question 10).

Over-provision of services is not assessed by the CANDID–S. The rating in these cases will depend on the underlying need rather than the services provided. Rate 1 (met need) if the respondent believes that a need is over-met by providing an additional service for an already met need; for example, providing day centre attendance in excess of what (in the respondent's view) is required. Rate 0 (no need) if a service is provided in an area of no need, for example psychiatric follow-up for a person who, in their view, does not need such support (Chapter 7, questions 8 & 9).

Recording CANDID–S assessments

The ratings can be recorded in the rating boxes of the CANDID–S itself. In order to minimise the possibility of the interviewer/rater being influenced by previous responses it may be preferable for each respondent's (user, carer, staff) views to be recorded on separate CANDID–S sheets.

Before starting the assessment, the user's name, the date of assessment and the assessor's initials are recorded in the box at the top of the page. Each assessment uses one of the three columns. Each of the 25 domains is then assessed.

At the end of the assessment, add up the number of domains with need rating 1 and record in row A (number of met needs). Add up the number domains with need rating 2 and record in row B (number of unmet needs). These two numbers are added to give the total number of domains in which a need has been assessed, and the sum is recorded in row C (total number of needs). Thus, three **summary scores** per interview can be calculated, giving a total maximum possible of nine if all respondents are interviewed.

5 Using the CANDID–R

What can CANDID–R be used for?

The CANDID–R (Appendix 2) is a semi-structured interview schedule for the assessment of needs of people with learning disabilities and mental health problems. It identifies needs (met and unmet) in 25 domains of life, as described in Chapter 3. In addition, it assesses the sources of help for the person and the respondent's satisfaction with services. It has been designed for research purposes.

The CANDID–R can be used as an audit or a research tool, along with other outcome measures, to evaluate the effectiveness of specific therapeutic interventions in people with learning disabilities and mental health problems. It can be used as a measure for research purposes, such as evaluating the impact on needs of two different types of mental health services or investigating the contribution of formal and informal carers in meeting needs. It can be used as a tool for planning services for people with learning disabilities at a population level (e.g. designing a service for a geographical area).

The CANDID–R schedule can also be used for interviewers using the CANDID–S (Chapter 4) to familiarise themselves with the full Section 1 for each domain. Inexperienced CANDID–S interviewers may find it helpful for the first few assessments to conduct the interview using Section 1 of the CANDID–R, while recording their ratings on the CANDID–S sheet. This is because some of the opening questions that appear in the CANDID–R have been omitted from the CANDID–S in order to keep it short.

Who can use CANDID–R?

Any person with experience in working with adults with learning disabilities and mental health problems can use CANDID–R. It can be completed by people from a variety of professional backgrounds including direct care workers, mental health professionals, social services practitioners, learning disabilities service planners, and researchers. Although the interviewer needs to have experience of clinical assessment interviews and previous experience of using assessment schedules is helpful, formal training is not a requirement for using CANDID–R. The interviewer should become familiar with the entire questionnaire before the first use. Subsequent assessments as well as interrater reliability are expected to improve by perusing this chapter. This book can be used as the basis for in-house training (Chapter 6) if, taking into account the local circumstances, this is thought to be useful, prior to introducing CANDID–R as a tool in a research project.

Whose views are assessed?

Three different perspectives can be assessed: those of the service *user* (patient, client, the person being assessed), informal *carer* (relative or friend) and *staff*. If an interview with the *user* is impossible, an advocate can be interviewed and instructed to answer the questions as if they were the user, rather than giving their own views. The informal *carer* can be anyone who is not paid for the care they provide. The *staff* respondent could be any member of staff who has a good knowledge of the person's circumstances, such as a direct care worker, a day centre staff member, a community nurse, a psychiatrist, etc.

A researcher interviews the user and informal carer, and either interviews the staff or gives a copy to the staff for self-completion. The assessments of user, carer and staff views can be in any order. Any of the three or all three assessments may be made

With the exception of an advocate responding on behalf of the person being assessed, respondents should be encouraged to give their own views on the needs of the user. It is this view (not the view of the interviewer) that is recorded. The perspectives of users, carers and staff may differ – this is why their assessments are recorded in different columns.

How is CANDID–R used?

The interview/assessment with each respondent uses one column. The assessment procedure in each domain is identical. The suggested questions, shown in italics, should be used to open discussion in each of the 25 domains. Additional questions should be asked keeping the purpose of each section in mind. The time frame used is the past **4 weeks** prior to the interview. Note that Sections 2, 3 and 4 are completed only if a need (met or unmet) has been identified in Section 1. Both subsections of Section 3 use the same set of anchor points.

To avoid confusion and repetition, each domain should be explored fully before questions about the next one are asked. However it is not essential that the order of domains is followed rigidly. Thus, if the respondent or the interviewer finds that, for example, *Inappropriate behaviour* follows naturally from *Safety of self*, asking questions in this order may be preferred. It is, of course, important that questions on all 25 domains are asked.

Each interview typically takes approximately 20–30 minutes to administer. This time becomes shorter as the interviewer becomes more familiar with using the scale. The duration of the interview, however, may vary, depending on the number of identified needs of the person being assessed and the respondent's attributes (e.g. interviewing an anxious parent or a distractible service user may prolong the duration of the interview). An explanation should be given prior to commencing the interview that its purpose is to identify rather than describe in detail each area of need.

Section 1

The definitions of met and unmet need in CANDID are based on the same principles as those adopted by the CAN (Slade *et al*, 1999).

A need is defined as met (need rating 1) when help is given for a particular problem and as a result of this, in the respondent's view:

a   the problem does not exist any more, OR

b   the problem is still present but only to a moderate degree, i.e. it does not constitute a serious problem any more.

A need in a particular domain is defined as unmet (need rating 2) if in the respondent's view:

a   there is a serious problem in this domain and no help is currently being given, OR

b   despite help there is still a serious problem.

Thus, there are four rating options based on the respondent's answers to the questions.

0=no need   no serious problem in this area & no help given
1=met need   no problem or only moderate problem due to help given
2=unmet need   serious problem exists whether or not help is given
9=not known   the respondent does not know the answer or does not want to answer.

If the problem persists despite any help that the person is receiving in this domain, then the distinction between met need and unmet need is a matter of judgement regarding the severity of the problem. The goal is to differentiate between problems that are current and serious, and those that are of moderate severity and are ameliorated by help. However, there may still be a blurred boundary where the user is receiving help, which only partly addresses their difficulties. It is the respondent's assessment of the degree of the problem that will guide the rating. A good question to identify the respondent's assessment is 'On balance, would you say that in this area there is a *serious problem*?' If the problem is only moderate or under control with the help the user is getting, then the need rating is 1 (met need), whereas if the problem is still considered to be current and serious, then the need rating is 2 (unmet need) (Chapter 7, question 7).

A response of 'no problem' requires further prompting to identify whether no problem exists because of help given (i.e. need rating 1 – met need), or no problem exists and no help is given (i.e. need rating 0 – no need). A rating of 1 is given if the reason for there being no problem is that the person is receiving help (i.e. there would be a problem if the help were to be withdrawn). A rating of 0 is given if the person is not receiving any help and still has no problem in this particular domain. A rating of 0 is also given if this domain does not apply to the user (see Chapter 7, question 1).

The CANDID–R makes no assumption that the reason for the existence of a need is the person's learning disability or mental health problems. Thus, if a person has not been able to use public transport in the past 4 weeks because of a physical illness, then the existence of a need in the Transport domain should be recorded and a rating of 1 or 2 should be given (see Chapter 7, question 10).

Over-provision of services is not assessed by the CANDID–R. The rating in these cases will depend on the underlying need rather than the services provided. Rate 1 (met need) if the respondent believes that a need is over-met by providing an additional service for an already met need; for example, providing day centre attendance in excess of what (in the respondent's view) is required. Rate 0 (no need) if a service is provided in an area of no need, for example psychiatric follow-up for a person who, in their view, does not need such support (Chapter 7, questions 8 & 9).

Section 2

This section assesses the help provided by informal sources, such as friends and family. There are five rating options:

0=no help   no helpful support is received in this area
1=low help   support received in this area is perceived as a little helpful
2=moderate help   support received in this area is perceived as quite helpful
3=high help   support received in this area is perceived as very helpful
9=not known

The rating key, complete with example anchor points to guide rating, is provided in a box following the relevant question in each domain. Note that there is no question about how much help the person needs from friends or relatives, only how much help is currently provided.

The purpose of this section is to record information about the current level of support for this domain from friends or family during the past 4 weeks. If the respondent has mentioned friends' names or family members, then the interviewer may personalise the question, but try not to exclude discussion of other people who might be helping. For example, *'Does your mum, or any other relative, help you to keep clean and tidy? How about friends?'* for Section 2 of Self-care.

The rating indicates the level of help received, and anchor points are provided for guiding the rating of level of help. Note that these are provided for guidance only and what is being rated is the respondent's perception of level of help. Thus, if the service user replied *'My dad talks to me when I feel sad, but he only makes things worse'* for the domain Other mental health problems, then this would be rated as 0 (no help). The same situation could be rated as 3 (high help) if at interview with the carer the response was *'I talk to him all the time when he is depressed, I think this helps him a lot'*. If both ratings were 3 (high help) on the basis of the same high level of input (frequency of visits), then the difference in the two perspectives would have been lost.

Commenting on the reported level of help is not recommended, as this could be perceived as either critical or patronising and may influence further responses. Also, it is the total level of help from (informal) sources that is being rated; it may be that help in different domains (or indeed in the same domain) is provided by different people.

Section 3

This section assesses the help provided by local services, such as a learning disability mental health team, social services, etc., and has two parts. Section 3a assesses the level of help currently being *provided* by local services, and Section 3b assesses how much help the respondent believes is *required*. There are five rating options. They are the same for both subsections and also identical to the rating options in Section 2.

The purpose of this section is to gain information about the current and required level of support from local services over the past month. The two parts are best asked separately. As with Section 2, the interviewer should attempt to personalise the questions by being specific about local services. For example, *'Do you talk to your keyworker here when you feel sad? Anyone else here?'* would be appropriate questions when interviewing a service user at a day centre.

For the first part of Section 3, as with Section 2, rating involves considering the effectiveness of an intervention, as perceived by the respondent. For example, if during the interview the user reports attending a day centre regularly, which he finds 'a waste of time', then the rating for help received (Section 3a) for *Daytime activities* should be 0 (no help). The examples with each rating are meant to show the type of intervention, which will constitute a low, medium or high level of help; what is being rated, however, is the level of perceived help.

The second part of Section 3 asks about the respondent's perception of the need for help. Try to emphasise the word 'need', rather than asking how much help the person would 'like' from local services. Note that the question is not asking how much extra help is needed. Use the same rating options as for the first part in this section. A rating of 0 would indicate that the respondent perceives no need for help from local services. When the same rating is given for the two subsections in this section, this may indicate an appropriate level of support from local services, or it may be that the right level but the wrong type of help is being given. When the rating is higher for the second question, this suggests the existence of unmet need: more help is needed than that currently received.

For both Sections 2 and 3, the rating reflects the help received or needed as judged by the respondent. Note that it is the respondent's views that are recorded, and not the interviewer's opinion as formed by the respondent's answers to the questions. The prompts given in the boxes are examples of what might be considered as low, moderate or high help on each occasion, and are provided for guidance only.

Section 4

There are two parts in Section 4. Section 4a asks about the respondent's view of the *appropriateness of the help* provided. Section 4b asks whether the respondent (other than a staff respondent) is satisfied with the *level of support* the person is receiving.

There are three rating options for each subsection:

0=not satisfied   overall the respondent is not satisfied with the help received from services
1=satisfied   overall the respondent is satisfied with the help received from services
9=not known

The two subsections' ratings may be different in cases where the respondent believes that the user is receiving a lot of help but of the wrong kind (e.g. counselling rather than medication for his or her mental health problems), or the right type of help but not enough of it (e.g. day centre attendance should be 5 rather than 2 days a week). Note that there is no question on staff satisfaction with the amount of help given by local services, to avoid conflict of interests.

The purpose of this section is to rate the respondent's perception of the appropriateness and effectiveness of interventions. It can be difficult to distinguish between the two questions in this section, but it may be that sometimes different ratings are given for the two questions. The first question asks about the appropriateness of the type of current interventions – do they think different help should be given? The second question asks (the user and carer only) about their satisfaction with the amount of help given – do they think more help should be given? Staff are not asked this question, since it could be seen as critical. This section is intended to identify when the person feels either the wrong type of help is being offered or not enough of the right type of help is being offered.

Recording CANDID–R assessments

CANDID–R ratings can be recorded directly in the boxes on the CANDID–R, in which case each interview uses one column. However, separate rating sheets (Appendix 3) for user, carer and staff ratings are also provided which can be used to record a CANDID–R assessment, one for each of the user, carer and staff interviews. In this case each interview/assessment uses one recording sheet. Their use minimises the risk of the interviewer's rating being influenced by previous interviews and reduces the amount of research datasheets to be stored.

In addition to individual domain ratings each rating sheet allows the recording of **summary scores,** which cannot be recorded directly onto the actual CANDID–R. These are:

i   three for Section 1: *Number of met needs* (add up the number of domains with need rating 1), *Number of unmet needs* (add up the number of domains with need rating 2), *Total number of needs* (*i.e.* the sum of met and unmet needs),

ii   one for Section 2: *Total level of help received from informal sources* (sum of Section 2 in all domains)

iii   two for Section 3: *Total level of help received from formal sources* (sum of Section 3a in all domains) and *Total level of help needed from formal sources* (sum of Section 3b in all domains),

iv   two for Section 4 (except for staff rating: only one): *Total level of satisfaction with type and amount of help* (no staff rating for Section 4b).

In adding up these totals, always count a need rating of 9 (not known) as 0.

6 Training for the CANDID

The CANDID–R and CANDID–S can be used by people with experience in clinical interviews without any formal training. Each version contains brief rating guidelines and in the CANDID–R every rating has anchor points for guidance. Whether using CANDID–S or CANDID–R, reading through the full CANDID–R will give the rater a good overview of the approach used, and a relatively good assessment can be expected from the first use.

There will, however, be times when some training in the use of the CANDID is appropriate. For example, if staff are not experienced in using standardised assessment scales, a training session may be used to increase familiarity and reduce the time taken to complete the questionnaire. If the CANDID–S is being introduced into routine clinical practice, there might be some resistance from staff, in which case training may serve to reduce apprehension, increase motivation and generate commitment from staff. If either version of the CANDID is planned to be used in a research project, training may be used to maximise inter-rater reliability from the outset.

This chapter provides an outline of a half-day training session. The length of the training session can be adjusted as required. The goal of this training is to educate participants about the approach taken to assessing needs and to give practice in rating the CANDID. As the principles underlying rating for the CANDID–R and CANDID–S are the same, the training can focus on either version or cover both. For CANDID–R training, the rating sheets provided in Appendix 3 are used to record ratings of the four sections. For CANDID–S training, only ratings from Section 1 are required and CANDID–S (Appendix 1) sheets are used for recording. The brief practice vignette (Appendix 5a) is used initially to familiarise participants with the rating procedure. Subsequently, the full vignette (Appendix 5b) can be used to assess needs in the 25 domains.

Each participant will need the following handouts:

1   Programme for the day
2   CANDID–S (Appendix 1) and/or CANDID–R (Appendix 2)
3   Brief practice vignette (Appendix 5a)
4   Full vignette (Appendix 5b)
5   CANDID–R rating sheets (Appendix 3)

The trainer will need an overhead projector, six overhead transparencies and a pen. The overheads for CANDID training can be photocopied from Appendix 4 and are as follows:

1   'Needs assessment in learning disabilities'
2   'CANDID: introduction'
3   'CANDID: need domains'
4   'CANDID–R: *Safety of others* assessment page'
5   'Met and unmet need: CANDID–R Section 1 or CANDID–S'
6   'Help and satisfaction: CANDID–R Sections 2, 3 & 4'

Overhead 6 is not required for CANDID–S training.

Introduction to needs assessment using CANDID (30 minutes)

Overhead: None
The trainer, after introducing him-/herself, may wish to go through the programme for the day, clarifying the time frame for each part of the training, break times, etc. Explain that the aim of the session is to introduce participants to the notion of need assessment and to give an outline of how to rate the CANDID. Emphasise that the format is one of a workshop rather than a lecture, and encourage participants to ask questions.

Overhead: 'Needs assessment in learning disabilities'
Using material material from Chapter 2:

- outline what a need is and why is it important to assess needs
- services should be provided on the basis of need
- everyone has needs, due to a variety of causes
- needs can be met or unmet
- the views of staff about need can differ from those of service users and their carers. It is important to note these differences.

Overhead: 'CANDID: introduction'
Using material material from Chapter 3:

- introduce CANDID
- brief history
- highlight principles & criteria for its development
- explain what purpose it will be used for locally.

Overhead: 'CANDID: need domains'

- introduce the 25 domains assessed by CANDID
- the domains cover a range of physical, mental health and social care needs
- every domain is assessed in the same way, so assessment is not as daunting as it might appear
- goal of training is to give confidence in rating, and to ensure agreement between raters.

Overhead: 'CANDID–R "Safety of others" assessment page' (use also for CANDID–S training)

- ask participants to find domain 15 in the CANDID–R
- introduce this as a typical page from the CANDID–R, stressing they are all structured the same way
- there are 4 sections in each domain, briefly explain what each rates
- notice that there are 3 columns for separate ratings by staff, user and carer, which are done in separate interviews
- it is acceptable for differences to exist between staff, carer and user ratings.

Overhead: 'Met and unmet need: CANDID–R Section 1 or CANDID–S'

- explain that CANDID–S assesses only Section 1 of the CANDID–R
- purpose of CANDID–R Section 1 or CANDID–S: to assess whether there is a problem in this domain
- use trigger questions (in italics in CANDID–R) to get into the topic
- always rate the response of the respondent
- define met and unmet need as described in Chapters 4 and 5

- introduce the concept of overmet need; CANDID does not measure it
- the anchor points provide just guidance for rating.

Overhead: 'Help and satisfaction: CANDID–R Sections 2, 3 & 4' (use only for CANDID–R training)

- Section 2 measures help received from informal sources – friends, relatives, neighbours, *etc.*
- Section 3 measures help received and needed from formal services
- level of help is being rated, with anchor points as guidance
- rate helpfulness of intervention, e.g. if an intervention is perceived as not helping at all, rate 0
- difference between help given and needed – stress the respondent's response is recorded
- highlight the difference between two parts of Section 4 (type vs. amount of help)

Although this overhead refers to CANDID–R only, it can be used for CANDID–S training in the interest of completeness.

Brief practice vignette (30–45 minutes) (Appendix 5a)

The goal is to have a first attempt at rating the CANDID, concentrating on a single domain through three brief role-play interviews. The expected ratings are given on a separate page in Appendix 5a. They can either be distributed with the vignette or after the participants have had the opportunity to role-play this particular part of an assessment interview:

- distribute vignette
- split into pairs, interviewer (rater) and John (patient, client, service user)
- emphasise that ratings are to be done in the 'User' column
- role-play interview for the assessment of *Safety of others* domain (5 minutes)
- stop the role-play, and discuss the scoring procedure in pairs (5 minutes)
- swap roles, so John becomes the interviewer/rater and the rater becomes the mother
- role-play assessment, emphasising that ratings are to be in the 'Carer' column (5 minutes)
- stop the role-play and discuss the scoring procedure in pairs (5 minutes)
- swap roles again: now the interviewer/rater interviews John's keyworker
- role-play assessment, emphasising that ratings are to be in the 'Staff' column (5 minutes)
- stop the role-play and discuss the scoring procedure in pairs (5 minutes).

Feedback on brief practice vignette (15–20 minutes)

Overhead: 'CANDID–R: "Safety of others" assessment page'
Go through the page, scoring on the overhead. If training for CANDID–S only, the trainer may emphasise that only Section 1 ratings from the three perspectives are required. In that case, the ratings can be recorded on the CANDID–S itself. However, it may be useful for participants to work through all four sections in order to get an overview of the rating approach. During the feedback the rating procedure in this domain is discussed, questions are encouraged and issues are addressed as they arise.

Full vignette (60 minutes) (Appendix 5b)

Distribute full vignette and completed assessment rating sheet
The rest of the programme can be tailored to individual requirements. Normally 1 hour is necessary for a full vignette. Different ways of running this part include:

1   In pairs, role-play the respondent (user or carer or staff) with the other one rating. This approach is useful for gaining familiarity with the CANDID–R, and generates most questions.

2   The trainer works through the vignette on the overhead projector, rating as he or she goes and inviting comments or alternative rating options on each rating. This approach is useful for a group lacking confidence in using assessment schedules.

3   The trainer role-plays the assessment with a volunteer (either could be the interviewer), while all participants rate from responses made. This approach is useful for participants seeing 'how to do it'.

7 Guidance on rating

Practical issues

Interviewing people with learning disabilities and mental health problems poses specific challenges. From the outset of the interview a brief introduction and explanation of the duration and purpose of the interview should be offered. This explanation might take the form: *'I'd like to ask you some questions using this form. This covers a number of areas of life in which people can have difficulties. I'll go through each of these areas and ask you if you had any problems in the last month. Please ask me if there is anything you do not undertand. Is that okay?'* The language used should reflect the level of learning disability of the person being interviewed. The interviewer should ensure that the person understands the question, and appropriate use of gestures, examples, rephrasing and repetition may be helpful. It is also important that the *answer* is understood correctly, and if there is uncertainty, the person should be asked to rephrase or explain his or her answer. If the respondent has specific communication difficulties, such as speech impediment in people with cerebral palsy or language idiosyncracies in people with autism, these should be noted and taken into account. The interviewer should also be aware of the tendency of some people with learning disabilities to be easily influenced (suggestibility) or agree with the person asking a question (acquiescence). Further prompting and clarification may be necessary, especially following 'closed' questions. As with any clinical contact, issues of *safety* and *confidentiality* should be observed.

Time should be allowed for questions, and to ensure that the assessment is not rushed. As discussed above, the assessment time will be affected by the number of needs identified and the characteristics of the respondent. The interview does not necessarily need to be completed in one session and it may be helpful or necessary to continue after a break, even on a different day.

Rating algorithm

In assessing the presence or absence of need (met or unmet), the need rating is made using the following algorithm. This applies to CANDID–R Section 1 and CANDID–S.

If the respondent does not know or does not want to answer the question,
    rate 9 (not known), *otherwise*
If a serious problem is present, irrespective of help given,
    rate 2 (unmet need), *otherwise*
If there is no serious problem
    rate 1 (met need), if this is because of help given, *or*
    rate 0 (no need), if no help is given

Frequently asked questions

This chapter contains a number of frequently asked questions that are equally applicable to CANDID–S and CANDID–R.

1. What should the need rating be if an area of need is not applicable (e.g. Basic education *in a profoundly disabled person*)?

'Not-applicable' does not exist as a rating option in CANDID. The absence (rating 0) or presence (rating 1 or 2) of need will be decided on the basis of the respondent's perception of existence of a serious problem and provision of help in this domain.

2. What if an intervention (e.g. counselling) is thought by the respondent to be necessary but is not available locally?

Local availability of an intervention is not a criterion for determining the existence of a need for this particular service. So if counselling for people with learning disabilities is not available locally but the respondent believes that it can help meet the person's need in a particular domain (e.g. *Other mental health problems*), then the need rating is *2* (unmet need).

3. Are depression and anxiety rated under Major mental health problems *or* Other mental health problems?

It depends on the severity of the mental health problems. If, in the respondent's view, the user's depression is severe enough to warrant specialist mental health care, then it is rated under *Major mental health problems*. Otherwise it is rated under *Other mental health problems*. For example, severe and disabling depressive and obsessive–compulsive conditions should be considered under *Major mental health problems*.

4. If the existence of a need has been identified in one area (e.g. difficulties with walking under Mobility), should it be rated under other relevant areas (e.g. difficulty with shopping and cooking under Food) as well?

Yes. Different needs may have the same cause. The CANDID makes no assumptions about the reason for the existence of a need. If a problem already rated under one area impacts on other areas and creates a need in more than one domain, then these needs should be rated separately. Once an unmet need is identified in any domain, further assessment may be necessary to decide on appropriate interventions. Please note specific exclusion clauses in rating domains 6 (*General physical health*) and 16 (*Inappropriate behaviour*).

5. In cases where a carer or member of staff is not familiar with certain aspects of the person's care, how do I rate responses like 'I don't know for sure, but I guess...'

If the respondent is not certain about the answer, then the need rating is *9* (*not known*).

6. If a person refuses to answer or it is obvious that their assessment is not accurate, can I correct the answer to reflect what is already known?

No. The ratings in each column must reflect the views of the respondent alone.

7. If a person is receiving help but the problem still exists, how is need rated?

The rating will depend on the respondent's perception of the impact the intervention has had on the problem. Rate 1 (met need) if the respondent believes that the problem has been alleviated significantly by the intervention, i.e. the problem currently is of a moderate degree or less. Rate 2 (unmet need) if the respondent believes that the intervention offered has not helped the problem at all or has helped only slightly, so that a serious problem still exists.

8. How is over-provision of services rated?

Over-provision of services is not assessed by CANDID. The rating in these cases will depend on the underlying need rather than the services that are over-provided. Rate 1 (met need) if the respondent believes that a need is over-met by providing an additional service in an area of met need. Rate 0 (no need) if a need is over-met by providing a service in an area of no need.
See also next question for an example of the two types of over-met need.

9. What is the need rating for Accommodation when the person has been an in-patient for more than a month?

Different rating options are appropriate according to circumstances. Rate 1 (met need) if the respondent believes that the person is appropriately placed in the hospital currently *or* if satisfactory accommodation is available on discharge. If both conditions apply, this is an over-met need (providing an additional service in an area of met need). Rate 2 (unmet need) if the respondent believes that being in hospital is not appropriate, and no alternative suitable accommodation is available. Rate 0 (no need) if although hospital accommodation is currently provided, this is not appropriate and the person has satisfactory accommodation outside hospital. This is another type of over-met need (providing a service in an area of no need).

10. If a person with learning disabilities is currently unable to look after his home due to physical health problems rather than because of his learning disabilities, then how do I rate the Looking after the home domain?

A need does not have to be due to the learning disabilities or the mental health problems in order to be rated. If there is currently a problem in this domain, then the existence of a need should be recorded by rating 1 (met need) or 2 (unmet need), depending on the seriousness of the problem.

11. What is the rating if there is currently no problem but only because of help given in the past? For example, if a person knows about his condition and treatment because of information that was given in the past, is Information need rated as 0 (no need) or 1 (met need)?

The rating will depend on whether the procedure for remedying the problem is currently in place. If the arrangements for giving information are ongoing (e.g. through a community nurse, users' group, etc.), then rate 1 (met need). If this was done in the past but not currently, rate 0 (no need).

Specific rating issues in each need domain

On rating each of the 25 domains, there are some specific issues that have been found to require clarification:

1. Accommodation

If a person is currently in hospital and does not have a home to be discharged to, the need rating is 1 (met need). If a person is currently in hospital and does have an appropriate home to be discharged to, the need rating is 0 (no need). The latter is an example of overmet need, which the CANDID does not assess.

2. Food

A need is present if the person is not getting an adequate diet, due to difficulties with shopping, storage and/or cooking of food, or because inadequate or inappropriate food is being provided (e.g. by a hospital ward). However, if the problem is primarily due to, for example, difficulties with budgeting, then this should be rated under the relevant domain (*Money budgeting*) and the *Food* rating should be 0.

3. Looking after the home

This domain concerns difficulties in maintaining the living environment, whether this is a group home room or an independent home. If not at home, this domain is rated in relation to the living environment that the person occupies at the time. If the person is homeless, the respondent may be able to state whether they believe it would be a problem if they had a home; if not, a rating of 9 (not known) is given.

4. Self-care

This domain refers to personal hygiene, and the person's cleanliness and tidiness. It does not include unusual or bizarre appearance.

5. Daytime activities

If the user is unable to occupy themselves during the day without help, then they have a need in this domain. Help given might include sheltered employment, attending a day centre, or activities with friends and relatives. If the primary problem is loneliness rather than inactivity and boredom, then this should be rated under the domain of *Social relationships*.

6. General physical health

Physical side-effects of medication should be considered, as well as any acute or chronic medical or dental condition. Do not include needs arising from specific sensory and mobility problems or epilepsy, as they are dealt with in domains 7, 8 and 9, respectively.

7. Eyesight/hearing

The use of a hearing aid or glasses implies automatically that a need is present; whether it is being met (need rating 1) or not (need rating 2) will depend on whether the respondent believes that the vision or hearing is adequately corrected with the help of the aids.

8. Mobility

Similarly to 7, if the person is, for example, wheelchair-bound but is able to move around because of adequate wheelchair access facilities and modifications in the living environment, then the need rating is 1 (met need). Otherwise it is 2 (unmet need).

9. Seizures

Problems with control of seizures and access to epilepsy clinics are rated here. Side-effects of anti-epileptic medication are also rated here.

10. Major mental health problems

When asking the user about this domain, particular care should be taken to record their perceptions. For example, a user who denies hearing voices and having problems with their thoughts, and states that their depot injection is to help them sleep, should be rated as 0 (no need).

11. Other mental health problems

This should include depression and anxiety of mild or moderate severity, regardless of the cause. However, severe depressive or anxiety states such as manic depressive illness and severe obsessive–compulsive disorder should be considered under domain 10.

12. Information

This should include information about local service provision, as well as information about the specific condition(s) the user has been diagnosed with, medication or other treatment he is receiving.

13. Exploitation risk

A wide range of vulnerability issues is covered here without a reference to the actual cause of the vulnerability (e.g. lack of skills due to learning disabilities or false beliefs due to mental health problems, etc).

14. Safety of self

Risk of suicide and self-harm caused either deliberately or inadvertently (e.g. road safety, severe self-neglect) are rated in this domain, but safety considerations due to vulnerability to exploitation are rated under domain 13.

15. Safety of others

Inadvertent risks (e.g. fire risk due to careless use of cigarettes) are included, as well as risk of deliberate violence, firesetting, etc. Risk to others arising from sexual behaviour is rated under domain 20 (*Sexual expression*).

16. Inappropriate behaviour

This includes socially embarrassing or objectionable behaviour, but not self-injurious, violent or sexually inappropriate behaviour, which are covered under domains 14, 15 and 20. 'Challenging behaviours' such as spitting, smearing, screaming, etc. are rated here.

17. Substance misuse

Alcohol and drug misuse is covered in this domain. Clarification questions should be asked to elicit possible misuse of illicit drugs, prescribed medication and non-prescribed medication.

18. Communication

This domain assesses both expressive and receptive (verbal and non-verbal) communication difficulties. Social aspects of communication (as for example in the case of people with autism) are also considered here.

19. Social relationships

Some of the daytime activities assessed in domain 5 may also facilitate social interaction, in addition to occupation. The two aspects should be enquired about separately and rated in the respective domain. One person (e.g. a friend) visiting may help meet the person need in the *Daytime activities* domain or *Social relationships* domain, or both.

20. Sexual expression

This includes difficulties in sexual function (including due to medication side-effects), as well as a lack of safe sex practices and inadequate contraception. Needs arising from inappropriate sexual expression, such as unacceptable sexual behaviour and sexual offending, are also included here.

21. Caring for someone else

For a need to be present the person being assessed does not have to be the sole or main carer. If it is perceived that the user has a caring role and receives or requires help with this, then a need is identified and the rating is 1 (met need) or 2 (unmet need).

22. Basic education

This question can trigger a 'not-applicable' response in the case of, for example, a profoundly disabled individual. A 'not-applicable' rating does not exist in CANDID. If the respondent believes that the user benefits or could benefit from education input currently, then the need rating is 1 (met need) or 2 (unmet need), depending on whether help is being received. If the respondent believes that this has been tried in the past and the person is not able to use help in this domain, then the need rating is 0 (no need).

23. Transport

A need is rated if the person has difficulties using public transport, whether for physical, psychological or social reasons. There may be overlap between this domain and the *Mobility* domain, but each need is rated separately.

24. Money budgeting

This refers to ability to cope with the available amount of money. If the user says they do not have enough money, this is assessed under *Welfare benefits*.

25. Welfare benefits

If a member of staff is not sure whether this domain is a need, but assumes that a colleague would have identified any need, then the need rating is 9 (not known).

References

Aman, M. G., Singh, N., Stewart, A. W., et al (1985) The Aberrant Behavior Checklist: A behavior rating scale for the assessment of treatment effects. *American Journal of Mental Deficiency*, **89**, 485–491.

Bailey, N. & Cooper, S-A. (1998) NHS beds for people with learning disabilities. *Psychiatric Bulletin*, **22**, 69–72.

Bouras, N. (1999) Mental health in learning disabilities: planning and service developments. *Tizard Learning Disability Review*, **4**, 3–5.

—— & Holt, G. (2001) Community mental health services for adults with learning disabilities. In *Textbook of Community Psychiatry* (eds G. Thornicroft & G. Szmukler), pp. 397–407. Oxford: Oxford University Press.

Bradshaw, J. (1972) A taxonomy of social need. In *Problems and Progress in Medical Care. Essays on Current Research* (ed. G. McLachlan). Oxford: Oxford University Press.

Department of Health (1997) *The New NHS: Modern, Dependable* (Cm 3807). London: Department of Health.

—— (1999a) *Modernising Mental Health Services*. London: Department of Health.

—— (1999b) *National Service Framework for Mental Health*. London: Department of Health.

—— (2001) *Valuing People: A New Strategy for Learning Disabilities for the 21st Century* (Cm5086). London: Department of Health.

Department of Health Social Services Inspectorate (1991) *Care Management and Assessment: Summary of Practice Guidance*. London: HMSO.

Doll, E. A. (1965) *The Vineland Social Maturity Scale*. Circle Pines, MN: American Guidance Service.

Eaton, I. F. & Menolascino, F. J. (1982) Psychiatric disorders in the mentally retarded. Types, problems and challenges. *American Journal of Psychiatry*, **139**, 1298–1303.

Gravestock, S. & Bouras, N. (1997) Survey of services for people with learning disabilities. *Psychiatric Bulletin*, **21**, 197–199.

Hassiotis, A., Barron, P. & O'Hara, J. (2000) Mental health services for people with learning disabilities. *British Medical Journal*, **321**, 583–584.

Holmes, N., Shah, A. & Wing, L. (1982) The Disability Assessment Schedule: A brief screening device for use with the mentally retarded. *Psychological Medicine*, **12**, 879–890.

House of Commons (1990) *The National Health Service and Community Care Act*. London: HMSO.

Jeffree, D. & Cheseldine, S. (1982) *Pathways to Independence. Checklists of Self-Help, Personal and Social Skills*. Northfleet: Stoneford Press.

Kazdin, A. E., Matson, J. L. & Senator, V. (1983) Assessment of depression in mentally retarded adults. *American Journal of Psychiatry*, **140**, 1040–1043.

McConkey, R. & Walsh, J. (1982) An index of social competence for use in determining the service needs of mentally handicapped people. *Journal of Mental Deficiency Research*, **26**, 47–61.

Mooney, G. (1986) Need, demand and the agency relationship. In *Economics, Medicine and Health Care* (ed G. Mooney). London: Harvester Wheatsheaf.

Moss, S., Prosser, H., Costello, H., et al (1998) Reliability and validity of the PAS–ADD Checklist for detecting psychiatric disorders in adults with intellectual disability. *Journal of Intellectual Disability Research*, **42**, 173–183.

Nihira, K., Foster, R., Shelhaas, M., et al (1974) *AAMD Adaptive Behavior Scale*. Washington, DC: American Association on Mental Deficiency.

O'Brien, G., Pearson, J., Berney, T., et al (2001) Measuring behaviour in developmental disability: a review of existing schedules. *Developmental Medicine and Child Neurology* (suppl. 87).

Orrell, M. & Hancock, G. (2004) *CANE: Camberwell Assessment of Need for the Elderly. A Needs Assessment for Older Mental Health Service Users*. London: Gaskell, in press.

Phelan, M., Slade, M., Thornicroft, G., et al (1995) The Camberwell Assessment of Need: The validity and reliability of an instrument to assess the needs of people with severe mental illness. *British Journal of Psychiatry*, **167**, 589–595.

Reiss, S. (1988) *The Reiss Screen for maladaptive behaviour test manual.* Chicago: International Diagnostic Systems.

— (1994) Psychopathology in mental retardation. In *Mental Health in Mental Retardation* (ed. N. Bouras). Cambridge: Cambridge University Press.

Royal College of Psychiatrists (1996) *Meeting the Mental Health Needs of Adults with Mild Learning Disabilities* (Council Report CR56). London: Royal College of Psychiatrists.

Shackleton-Bailey, M. J. & Pidcock, B. E. (1983) *Hampshire Assessment of Living with Others (5th version).* Winchester: Hampshire Social Services.

Slade, M. (1994) Needs assessment: involvement of staff and users will help to meet needs. *British Journal of Psychiatry,* **165**, 293–296.

—, Thornicroft, G., Loftus, L., *et al* (1999) *CAN: The Camberwell Assessment of Need.* London: Gaskell.

Sovner, R. & Hurley, A. D. (1983) Do the mentally retarded suffer from affective illness? *Archives of General Psychiatry,* **40**, 61–67.

Stevens, A. & Gabbay, J. (1991) Needs assessment needs assessment. *Health Trends,* **23**, 20–23.

Thomas, S., Harty, M.-A., Parrott, J., *et al* (2003) *CANFOR: Camberwell Assessment of Need – Forensic Version. A Needs Assessment for Forensic Mental Health Service Users.* London: Gaskell.

Thornicroft, G. (2000) National Service Framework for Mental Health. *Psychiatric Bulletin,* **24**, 203–206.

White, M. J., Nichols, C. N., Cook, R. S., *et al* (1995) Diagnostic overshadowing and mental retardation: a meta-analysis. *American Journal of Mental Retardation,* **100**, 293–298.

Williams, C. (1982) *The STAR Profile: Social Training Achievement Record.* Kidderminster: British Institute of Mental Handicap.

Xenitidis, K., Thornicroft, G., Leese, M., *et al* (2000) Reliability and validity of the CANDID – a needs assessment instrument for adults with learning disabilities and mental health problems. *British Journal of Psychiatry,* **176**, 473–478.

Appendix 1

Camberwell Assessment of Need for Adults with Developmental and Intellectual Disabilities – Short Version (CANDID–S)

How to use CANDID–S

What is CANDID–S?

The *Camberwell Assessment of Need for Adults with Developmental and Intellectual Disabilities* (CANDID) is a needs assessment scale specifically designed for people with learning disabilities and mental health problems. CANDID was developed at the Institute of Psychiatry, London, by modification of the *Camberwell Assessment of Need* (CAN), an established needs assessment scale for people with severe mental illness. The validity and reliability of CANDID have been investigated in community and hospital settings and were found to be acceptable (Xenitidis *et al*, 2000).

CANDID–S (Short version) is a brief (one-page) semi-structured interview schedule screening need in 25 life domains. It aims to establish i) if there is a need in each of these domains, and ii) if a need exists, whether it is currently met or unmet.

CANDID–R (Research version) addresses in addition the issues of who is each need met by (professional or informal sources) and whether the respondent is satisfied with the help the person is getting.

Who can complete CANDID–S?

CANDID–S is completed by the person conducting the interview. It can be completed by people from a variety of professional backgrounds. Although the interviewer needs to have experience of clinical assessment interviews, no formal training is required.

Who should be interviewed?

The interviewer may choose to interview the service *user* (the person being assessed), an informal *carer* (relative or friend) or a *staff* member who knows the user sufficiently well. Any of the three or all three may be interviewed and their perspectives may differ; this is why they are recorded in different columns. If an interview with the *user* is not possible, an advocate should be interviewed and instructed to answer the questions as if they were the user, rather than giving their own views. The *carer* can be a relative or a friend, generally someone who is not paid for the care they provide. The *staff* interview can be with any member of staff who has a good knowledge of the person's circumstances.

How is CANDID–S completed?

Each interview uses one column. The suggested questions, shown in italics, should be used to open discussion in each of the 25 domains. Additional questions should be asked with the goal of establishing whether the user has a need (currently met or unmet) in this domain. The time-scale used is the past 4 weeks prior to the interview.

How is CANDID–S rated?

0 = no need	indicates that there is no serious problem or difficulty in this area
1 = met need	indicates that because of help given, the person has no problem or has only a moderate problem in this area
2 = unmet need	indicates that a serious problem exists in this area, whether or not help is given
9 = not known	indicates that the person interviewed does not know about the particular domain or does not wish to disclose any information about any problems/ difficulties that they know about.

If the problem persists despite help, it is the respondent's assessment of the degree of the problem that determines the rating: 1 (met need) if the problem is only moderate or 2 (unmet need) if it is serious.

Over-provision of services is not assessed by CANDID. The rating should be 1 (met need) or 0 (no need), reflecting the underlying need.

A response of 'no problem' requires further prompting to distinguish between no need (0) and met need (1).

Please refer to Chapters 4, 6 and 7 for full instructions, frequently asked questions and worked examples of needs assessment using CANDID–S.

CANDID–S

| User name _____ | 0 = No need | 1 = Met need |
| Date of assessment __ / __ / __ Initials of assessor _____ | 2 = Unmet need | 9 = Not known |

		User	Carer	Staff
1.	**Accommodation** *What kind of place do you live in? Do you have any problems with it?*			
2.	**Food** *Do you get enough to eat? Do you make your own meals?*			
3.	**Looking after the home** *Are you able to look after your home or room? Does anyone help you?*			
4.	**Self-care** *Do you have any problems keeping yourself clean and tidy? Do you need reminding or help?*			
5.	**Daytime activities** *How do you spend your day? Do you have enough to do during the day?*			
6.	**General physical health** (excluding specific problems rated in domains 7, 8 & 9) *Do you have any health problems? Are you getting any treatment for physical problems?*			
7.	**Eyesight/hearing** *Do you have any problems with eyesight or hearing? Do you use a hearing aid or glasses?*			
8.	**Mobility** *Do you have difficulty moving about inside or outside the home?*			
9.	**Seizures** *Do you ever get fits? Are you getting any treatment for them?*			
10.	**Major mental health problems** *Do you ever hear voices or have problems with your thoughts?*			
11.	**Other mental health problems** *Have you recently felt very sad or low? Have you felt overly anxious or frightened?*			
12.	**Information** *Has anybody explained to you about your condition and treatment?*			
13.	**Exploitation risk** *Is anyone trying to take advantage of you? Can you stand up for yourself?*			
14.	**Safety of self** *Have you ever had thoughts of harming yourself? Do you do anything to put yourself at risk?*			
15.	**Safety of others** *Do you ever lose your temper and hit people? Do you think you can be a danger to others?*			
16.	**Inappropriate behaviour** (excluding specific problems rated in domains 14, 15 & 20) *Do other people get annoyed, upset or angry because of your behaviour?*			
17.	**Substance misuse** *Does drinking alcohol cause you any problems? Do you take drugs that are not prescribed?*			
18.	**Communication** *Can you understand what other people say to you? Can they understand you?*			
19.	**Social relationships** *Do you have enough friends? Do you wish you had more contact with people?*			
20.	**Sexual expression** *Do you have any sexual difficulties?*			
21.	**Caring for someone else** *Do you have any children under 18 or a relative you are looking after?*			
22.	**Basic education** *Do you have difficulty in reading and writing? Can you count your change in a shop?*			
23.	**Transport** *Can you travel by bus, tube or train? Do you get a free bus pass?*			
24.	**Money budgeting** *How do you find budgeting your money? Do you get help with things such as paying your bills?*			
25.	**Welfare benefits** *Are you sure you are getting all the money you are entitled to?*			

	User	Carer	Staff
A – Met needs (count the number of 1s in the column)			
B – Unmet needs (count the number of 2s in the column)			
C – Total number of needs (add together A and B)			

Contents

1 Accommodation

Assessments

| User rating | Carer rating | Staff rating |

Does the person lack a current appropriate place to live?

What kind of place do you live in?
Do you have any problems with your house, flat or room?

CAN0101 CAN0102 CAN0103

Rating	Meaning	Example
0	No need	The person has an adequate home (even if in hospital)
1	Met need	The person is living in sheltered or residential accommodation
2	Unmet need	The person is homeless or lacks basic facilities such as water and electricity
9	Not known	

If rated 0 or 9 go to Question 2

How much help does the person receive from friends or relatives with their accommodation?

CAN0104 CAN0105 CAN0106

Rating	Meaning	Example
0	None	
1	Low help	Occasionally supplied with items of furniture
2	Moderate help	Substantial help with improving accommodation, such as redecoration of flat
3	High help	Living with relative because own accommodation is unsatisfactory
9	Not known	

How much help does the person *receive* from local services with their accommodation?

CAN0107 CAN0108 CAN0109

How much help does the person *need* from local services with their accommodation?

CAN0110 CAN0111 CAN0112

Rating	Meaning	Example
0	None	
1	Low help	Minor decoration, was given address of housing agency
2	Moderate help	Major improvements, referral to housing agency
3	High help	Being rehoused, living in group home or hostel
9	Not known	

Does the person receive the right type of help with their accommodation?

CAN0113 CAN0114 CAN0115

(0=No; 1=Yes; 9=Not known)

Overall, is the respondent satisfied with the amount of help the person is receiving with their accommodation?

CAN0116 CAN0117

(0=Not satisfied; 1=Satisfied; 9=Not known)

2 Food

Does the person have difficulty in getting enough food?

Do you get enough to eat?
Do you make your own meals? Do you do your own shopping?

CAN0201   CAN0202   CAN0203

Rating	Meaning	Example
0	No need	Able to buy and prepare meals
1	Met need	Unable to prepare food and has meals provided
2	Unmet need	Very restricted diet, inappropriate food
9	Not known	

If rated 0 or 9 go to Question 3

How much help does the person receive from friends or relatives with getting enough to eat?

CAN0204   CAN0205   CAN0206

Rating	Meaning	Example
0	None	
1	Low help	Meals provided weekly or less often
2	Moderate help	Help with shopping or meals provided more than weekly but less than daily
3	High help	Meals provided daily
9	Not known	

How much help does the person *receive* from local services with getting enough to eat?

CAN0207   CAN0208   CAN0209

How much help does the person *need* from local services with getting enough to eat?

CAN0210   CAN0211   CAN0212

Rating	Meaning	Example
0	None	
1	Low help	1–4 meals a week provided, or assisted for one meal a day
2	Moderate help	More than 4 meals a week provided, or assisted for all meals
3	High help	All meals provided
9	Not known	

Does the person receive the right type of help with getting enough to eat?

CAN0213   CAN0214   CAN0215

(0=No; 1=Yes; 9=Not known)

Overall, is the respondent satisfied with the amount of help the person is receiving in getting enough to eat?

CAN0216   CAN0217

(0=Not satisfied; 1=Satisfied; 9=Not known)

3 Looking after the home

Does the person have difficulty looking after the home?

CAN0301 CAN0302 CAN0303

Are you able to look after your home?
Does anyone help you with keeping your home/flat/room tidy?

Rating	Meaning	Example
0	No need	Home may be untidy but the person keeps it basically clean
1	Met need	Unable to look after home and has regular domestic help
2	Unmet need	Home is dity and a potential health hazard
9	Not known	

If rated 0 or 9 go to Question 4

How much help does the person receive from friends or relatives with looking after the home?

CAN0304 CAN0305 CAN0306

Rating	Meaning	Example
0	None	
1	Low help	Prompts or helps tidy up or clean occasionally
2	Moderate help	Prompts or helps clean at least once a week
3	High help	Supervises the person more than once a week, washes all clothes and cleans the home
9	Not known	

How much help does the person *receive* from local services with looking after the home?

CAN0307 CAN0308 CAN0309

How much help does the person *need* from local services with looking after the home?

CAN0310 CAN0311 CAN0312

Rating	Meaning	Example
0	None	
1	Low help	Prompting by staff
2	Moderate help	Some assistance with household tasks
3	High help	Majority of household tasks done by staff
9	Not known	

Does the person receive the right type of help with looking after the home?

CAN0313 CAN0314 CAN0315

(0=No; 1=Yes; 9=Not known)

Overall, is the respondent satisfied with the amount of help the person is receiving in looking after the home?

CAN0316 CAN0317

(0=Not satisfied; 1=Satisfied; 9=Not known)

4 Self-care

Assessments

User rating   Carer rating   Staff rating

Does the person have difficulty with self-care?

CAN0401 CAN0402 CAN0403

Do you have problems keeping yourself clean and tidy?
Do you ever need reminding or help? Who by?

Rating	Meaning	Example
0	No need	Appearance may be unusual, eccentric or untidy, but basically clean
1	Met need	Needs and gets help with self-care
2	Unmet need	Poor personal hygiene, person smells
9	Not known	

If rated 0 or 9 go to Question 5

How much help does the person receive from friends or relatives with their self-care?

CAN0404 CAN0405 CAN0406

Rating	Meaning	Example
0	None	
1	Low help	Occasionally prompt the person to change their clothes
2	Moderate help	Run the bath/shower and insist on its use, daily prompting
3	High help	Provide daily assistance with several aspects of care
9	Not known	

How much help does the person *receive* from local services with their self-care?

CAN0407 CAN0408 CAN0409

How much help does the person *need* from local services with their self-care?

CAN0410 CAN0411 CAN0412

Rating	Meaning	Example
0	None	
1	Low help	Occasional prompting
2	Moderate help	Supervise weekly washing
3	High help	Supervise several aspects of self-care, self-care skills programme
9	Not known	

Does the person receive the right type of help with self-care?

CAN0413 CAN0414 CAN0415

(0=No; 1=Yes; 9=Not known)

Overall, is the respondent satisfied with the amount of help the person is receiving with self-care?

CAN0416 CAN0417

(0=Not satisfied; 1=Satisfied; 9=Not known)

5 Daytime activities

Does the person have difficulty with regular, appropriate daytime activities?

CAN0501 CAN0502 CAN0503

How do you spend your day?
Do you have enough to do during the day?

Rating	Meaning	Example
0	No need	In full-time employment, or adequately occupied with household/social activities
1	Met need	Unable to occupy self, so attending day centre
2	Unmet need	No employment of any kind and not adequately occupied with household or social activities
9	Not known	

If rated 0 or 9 go to Question 6

How much help does the person receive from friends or relatives in finding or keeping regular and appropriate daytime activities?

CAN0504 CAN0505 CAN0506

Rating	Meaning	Example
0	None	
1	Low help	Occasional advice about daytime activities
2	Moderate help	Has arranged daytime activities such as adult education or day centre attendance
3	High help	Daily help with arranging daytime activities
9	Not known	

How much help does the person *receive* from local services with their daytime activities?

CAN0507 CAN0508 CAN0509

How much help does the person *need* from local services with their daytime activities?

CAN0510 CAN0511 CAN0512

Rating	Meaning	Example
0	None	
1	Low help	Employment training/adult education
2	Moderate help	Sheltered employment daily. Day centre 2–4 days/week
3	High help	Attends day hospital or day centre daily
9	Not known	

Does the person receive the right type of help with daytime activities?

CAN0513 CAN0514 CAN0515

(0=No; 1=Yes; 9=Not known)

Overall, is the respondent satisfied with the amount of help the person is receiving with daytime activities?

CAN0516 CAN0517

(0=Not satisfied; 1=Satisfied; 9=Not known)

6 General physical health

Assessments
User   Carer   Staff
rating   rating   rating

Does the person have any physical illness or any drug side-effects? (exclude specific problems rated under domains 7, 8 & 9)

Do you have any problems with your physical health (e.g. chest, stomach etc.)?
Are you getting any treatment for physical health problems from your doctor?

CAN0601 CAN0602 CAN0603

Rating	Meaning	Example
0	No need	Physically well, within the constraints of any long-standing physical impairment
1	Met need	Physical ailment, such as high blood pressure, receiving appropriate treatment
2	Unmet need	Untreated physical ailment, including side-effects
9	Not known	

If rated 0 or 9 go to Question 7

How much help does the person receive from friends or relatives for physical health problems?

CAN0604 CAN0605 CAN0606

Rating	Meaning	Example
0	None	
1	Low help	Prompting to go to the doctor
2	Moderate help	Accompanied to doctor
3	High help	Daily help with physical health problems
9	Not known	

How much help does the person *receive* from local services for physical health problems?

CAN0607 CAN0608 CAN0609

How much help does the person *need* from local services for physical health problems?

CAN0610 CAN0611 CAN0612

Rating	Meaning	Example
0	None	
1	Low help	Given dietary or other health advice
2	Moderate help	Prescribed medication. Regularly seen by GP/nurse
3	High help	Frequent hospital appointments
9	Not known	

Does the person receive the right type of help for physical problems?

CAN0613 CAN0614 CAN0615

(0=No; 1=Yes; 9=Not known)

Overall, is the respondent satisfied with the amount of help the person is receiving for physical problems?

CAN0616 CAN0617

(0=Not satisfied; 1=Satisfied; 9=Not known)

7 Eyesight/hearing

Does the person have any problems with seeing or hearing?

Do you have difficulty in hearing what someone is saying?
Can you see well? (e.g. newspaper, television, etc.)

CAN0701   CAN0702   CAN0703

Rating	Meaning	Example
0	No need	Can see and hear well without aids
1	Met need	Hearing aid/spectacles required
2	Unmet need	Very poor eyesight/hearing
9	Not known	

If rated 0 or 9 go to Question 8

How much help does the person receive from friends or relatives with their eyesight/hearing problems?

CAN0704   CAN0705   CAN0706

Rating	Meaning	Example
0	None	
1	Low help	Prompting to seek help or advice
2	Moderate help	Accompanies to appointments, helps with getting aids
3	High help	Accompanies almost everywhere outside the house
9	Not known	

How much help does the person *receive* from local services with their eyesight/hearing problems?

CAN0707   CAN0708   CAN0709

How much help does the person *need* from local services with their eyesight/hearing problems?

CAN0710   CAN0711   CAN0712

Rating	Meaning	Example
0	None	
1	Low help	Advice and minimal support
2	Moderate help	Aids provided. Medical investigations. Some assistance with tasks
3	High help	Assistance several days a week. Frequent hospital appointments
9	Not known	

Does the person receive the right type of help with their eyesight/hearing problems?

(0=No; 1=Yes; 9=Not known)

CAN0713   CAN0714   CAN0715

Overall, is the respondent satisfied with the amount of help the person is receiving with their eyesight/hearing problems?

(0=Not satisfied; 1=Satisfied; 9=Not known)

CAN0716   CAN0717

8 Mobility

Does the person have restricted mobility?

CAN0801 CAN0802 CAN0803

Do you have difficulty moving about inside or outside the house?
Do you need any help?

Rating	Meaning	Example
0	No need	Able to walk unaided
1	Met need	Mobile with some assistance/aids
2	Unmet need	Not mobile
9	Not known	

If rated 0 or 9 go to Question 9

How much help does the person receive from friends or relatives with their mobility problems?

CAN0804 CAN0805 CAN0806

Rating	Meaning	Example
0	None	
1	Low help	Occasional help. Prompts to seek help
2	Moderate help	Regularly accompanies on visits. Weekly help Some home alterations
3	High help	Help several times a week. Considerable home alterations
9	Not known	

How much help does the person *receive* from local services with their mobility problems?

CAN0807 CAN0808 CAN0809

How much help does the person *need* from local services with their mobility problems?

CAN0810 CAN0811 CAN0812

Rating	Meaning	Example
0	None	
1	Low help	Receives advice and aids
2	Moderate help	Regularly seen by physiotherapist/nurse. Weekly assistance. Some home alterations
3	High help	Assistance several times a week. Considerable home alterations
9	Not known	

Does the person receive the right type of help with their mobility problems?

CAN0813 CAN0814 CAN0815

(0=No; 1=Yes; 9=Not known)

Overall, is the respondent satisfied with the amount of help the person is receiving with their mobility problems?

CAN0816 CAN0817

(0=Not satisfied; 1=Satisfied; 9=Not known)

9 Seizures

Assessments

User rating	Carer rating	Staff rating

Does the person have any kind of seizures?

CAN0901 CAN0902 CAN0903

Do you ever get fits of any kind?
Are you getting any treatment from your doctor?

Rating	Meaning	Example
0	No need	No seizures. No anti-epileptic medication
1	Met need	Well-controlled epilepsy. On regular anti-epileptic medication
2	Unmet need	Frequent seizures
9	Not known	

If rated 0 or 9 go to Question 10

How much help does the person receive from friends or relatives for their seizures?

CAN0904 CAN0905 CAN0906

Rating	Meaning	Example
0	None	
1	Low help	Some supervision of medication
2	Moderate help	Regular supervision of medication
3	High help	Constant supervision of medication and help with seizures
9	Not known	

How much help does the person *receive* from local services for their seizures?

CAN0907 CAN0908 CAN0909

How much help does the person *need* from local services for their seizures?

CAN0910 CAN0911 CAN0912

Rating	Meaning	Example
0	None	
1	Low help	Seizures monitored by GP only
2	Moderate help	Seizures occasionally monitored by specialist services and infrequent nurse visits
3	High help	Frequent out-patient appointments or hospital admissions. Frequent specialist nurse visits
9	Not known	

Does the person receive the right type of help for their seizures?

CAN0913 CAN0914 CAN0915

(0=No; 1=Yes; 9=Not known)

Overall, is the respondent satisfied with the amount of help the person is receiving for their seizures?

CAN0916 CAN0917

(0=Not satisfied; 1=Satisfied; 9=Not known)

10 Major mental health problems

Does the person have any symptoms of severe mental illness?

Do you ever hear voices or have problems with your thoughts?
Are you on any medication or injections? What is it for?

CAN1001 CAN1002 CAN1003

Rating	Meaning	Example
0	No need	No positive symptoms, not at risk from symptoms and not on medication
1	Met need	Symptoms helped by medication or other help
2	Unmet need	Currently has symptoms or is at risk
9	Not known	

If rated 0 or 9 go to Question 11

How much help does the person receive from friends or relatives for these problems?

CAN1004 CAN1005 CAN1006

Rating	Meaning	Example
0	None	
1	Low help	Some sympathy and support
2	Moderate help	Carers involved in helping with coping strategies or medication compliance
3	High help	Constant supervision of medication and help with coping strategies
9	Not known	

How much help does the person *receive* from local services for these mental health problems?

CAN1007 CAN1008 CAN1009

How much help does the person *need* from local services for these mental health problems?

CAN1010 CAN1011 CAN1012

Rating	Meaning	Example
0	None	
1	Low help	Medication reviewed 3-monthly or less, support group
2	Moderate help	Medication reviewed more than 3-monthly, structured psychological therapy
3	High help	Medication and 24-hour hospital care or crisis care at home
9	Not known	

Does the person receive the right type of help for these mental health problems?

CAN1013 CAN1014 CAN1015

(0=No; 1=Yes; 9=Not known)

Overall, is the respondent satisfied with the amount of help the person is receiving for these problems?

CAN1016 CAN1017

(0=Not satisfied; 1=Satisfied; 9=Not known)

11 Other mental health problems

Does the person suffer from current psychological distress, anxiety or depression?

Have you recently felt very sad or low?
Have you felt overly anxious or frightened?

CAN1101 CAN1102 CAN1103

Rating	Meaning	Example
0	No need	Occasional or mild distress
1	Met need	Needs and gets ongoing support
2	Unmet need	Distress affects life significantly, such as preventing person going out
9	Not known	

If rated 0 or 9 go to Question 12

How much help does the person receive from friends or relatives for this distress?

CAN1104 CAN1105 CAN1106

Rating	Meaning	Example
0	None	
1	Low help	Some sympathy and support
2	Moderate help	Has opportunity at least weekly to talk about distress to a friend or relative
3	High help	Constant support and supervision
9	Not known	

How much help does the person *receive* from local services for this distress?

CAN1107 CAN1108 CAN1109

How much help does the person *need* from local services for this distress?

CAN1110 CAN1111 CAN1112

Rating	Meaning	Example
0	None	
1	Low help	Assessment of mental state or occasional support
2	Moderate help	Specific psychological or social treatment for anxiety. Counselled by staff at least once a week
3	High help	24-hour hospital care or crisis care
9	Not known	

Does the person receive the right type of help for these mental health problems?

CAN1113 CAN1114 CAN1115

(0=No; 1=Yes; 9=Not known)

Overall, is the respondent satisfied with the amount of help the person is receiving for these problems?

CAN1116 CAN1117

(0=Not satisfied; 1=Satisfied; 9=Not known)

12 Information (on condition and treatment)

Has the person had clear verbal or written information about their condition and treatment?

CAN1201 CAN1202 CAN1203

Has anybody explained to you why you need to see the doctor and have tablets or other treatment? Who did? Did you understand this?

Rating	Meaning	Example
0	No need	Has received and understood adequate information
1	Met need	Has not received or understood all information
2	Unmet need	Has received no information
9	Not known	

If rated 0 or 9 go to Question 13

How much help does the person receive from friends or relatives in obtaining such information?

CAN1204 CAN1205 CAN1206

Rating	Meaning	Example
0	None	
1	Low help	Has had some advice from friends or relatives
2	Moderate help	Given leaflets/fact sheets or put in touch with self-help groups by friends or relatives
3	High help	Regular liaison with doctors or groups such as MENCAP by friends or relatives
9	Not known	

How much help does the person *receive* from local services in obtaining such information?

CAN1207 CAN1208 CAN1209

How much help does the person *need* from local services in obtaining such information?

CAN1210 CAN1211 CAN1212

Rating	Meaning	Example
0	None	
1	Low help	Brief verbal or written information on illness/problem/treatment
2	Moderate help	Given details of self-help groups. Long verbal information sessions on drugs and alternatives
3	High help	Given detailed written information or has had specific personal edcation
9	Not known	

Does the person receive the right type of help in obtaining information?

CAN1213 CAN1214 CAN1215

(0=No; 1=Yes; 9=Not known)

Overall, is the respondent satisfied with the amount of help the person is receiving in obtaining information?

CAN1216 CAN1217

(0=Not satisfied; 1=Satisfied; 9=Not known)

13 Exploitation risk

User rating	Carer rating	Staff rating

Is the person at risk of being exploited or abused?

Is anyone trying to take advantage of you in any way (e.g. taking money off you or making you do sexual or other things that you don't want to do). Can you stand up for yourself and protect yourself or do you need help with this?

CAN1301 CAN1302 CAN1303

Rating	Meaning	Example
0	No need	Not vulnerable to exploitation/abuse
1	Met need	Needs and gets ongoing support and protection
2	Unmet need	Subject of regular verbal abuse, any financial misappropriation, physical or sexual abuse
9	Not known	

If rated 0 or 9 go to Question 14

How much help does the person receive from friends or relatives to reduce the risk of exploitation/abuse?

CAN1304 CAN1305 CAN1306

Rating	Meaning	Example
0	None	
1	Low help	Able to contact friends or relatives if feeling vulnerable
2	Moderate help	Friends or relatives are usually in contact and are likely to know if feeling vulnerable
3	High help	Friends or relatives in regular contact and are very likely to know and provide help if feeling vulnerable
9	Not known	

How much help does the person *receive* from local services to reduce the risk of exploitation/abuse?

CAN1307 CAN1308 CAN1309

How much help does the person *need* from local services to reduce the risk of exploitation/abuse?

CAN1310 CAN1311 CAN1312

Rating	Meaning	Example
0	None	
1	Low help	Someone to contact when feeling vulnerable
2	Moderate help	Regular monitoring and support
3	High help	Constant supervision, legal involvement via services
9	Not known	

Does the person receive the right type of help to reduce the risk of exploitation/abuse?

CAN1313 CAN1314 CAN1315

(0=No; 1=Yes; 9=Not known)

Overall, is the respondent satisfied with the amount of help the person is receiving to reduce the risk of exploitation/abuse?

CAN1316 CAN1317

(0=Not satisfied; 1=Satisfied; 9=Not known)

14 Safety of self

Is the person a danger to themselves?

Do you ever have thoughts of harming yourself? Do you ever actually harm yourself? Do you put yourself in danger in any way?

CAN1401 CAN1402 CAN1403

Rating	Meaning	Example
0	No need	No suicidal thoughts. No self-injury
1	Met need	Suicide/self-injury risk monitored by staff, receiving counselling
2	Unmet need	Has expressed suicidal ideas during past month or has exposed themselves to serious danger
9	Not known	

If rated 0 or 9 go to Question 15

How much help does the person receive from friends or relatives to reduce the risk of self-harm?

CAN1404 CAN1405 CAN1406

Rating	Meaning	Example
0	None	
1	Low help	Able to contact friends or relatives if feeling unsafe
2	Moderate help	Friends or relatives are usually in contact and are likely to know if feeling unsafe
3	High help	Friends or relatives in regular contact and are very likely to know and provide help if feeling unsafe
9	Not known	

How much help does the person *receive* from local services to reduce the risk of self-harm?

CAN1407 CAN1408 CAN1409

How much help does the person *need* from local services to reduce the risk of self-harm?

CAN1410 CAN1411 CAN1412

Rating	Meaning	Example
0	None	
1	Low help	Someone to contact when feeling unsafe
2	Moderate help	Staff check at least once a week, regular supportive counselling
3	High help	Daily supervision, in-patient care
9	Not known	

Does the person receive the right type of help to reduce the risk of self-harm?

CAN1413 CAN1414 CAN1415

(0=No; 1=Yes; 9=Not known)

Overall, is the respondent satisfied with the amount of help the person is receiving to reduce the risk of self-harm?

CAN1416 CAN1417

(0=Not satisfied; 1=Satisfied; 9=Not known)

15 Safety of others

Assessments

User rating	Carer rating	Staff rating

Is the person a current or potential risk to other peoples' safety?

Do you think you could be a danger to other people?
Do you ever lose your temper and hit people?

CAN1501	CAN1502	CAN1503

Rating	Meaning	Example
0	No need	No history of violence or threatening behaviour
1	Met need	Under supervision because of potential risk
2	Unmet need	Recent violence or threats
9	Not known	

If rated 0 or 9 go to Question 16

How much help does the person receive from friends or relatives to reduce the risk that they might harm someone else?

CAN1504	CAN1505	CAN1506

Rating	Meaning	Example
0	None	
1	Low help	Help with threatening behaviour weekly or less
2	Moderate help	Help with threatening behaviour more than weekly
3	High help	Almost constant help with persistently threatening behaviour
9	Not known	

How much help does the person *receive* from local services to reduce the risk that they might harm someone else?

CAN1507	CAN1508	CAN1509

How much help does the person *need* from local services to reduce the risk that they might harm someone else?

CAN1510	CAN1511	CAN1512

Rating	Meaning	Example
0	None	
1	Low help	Check on behaviour weekly or less
2	Moderate help	Daily supervision
3	High help	Constant supervision, anger management programme
9	Not known	

Does the person receive the right type of help to reduce the risk that they might harm someone else?

CAN1513	CAN1514	CAN1515

(0=No; 1=Yes; 9=Not known)

Overall, is the respondent satisfied with the amount of help the person is receiving to reduce the risk that they might harm someone else?

CAN1516	CAN1517

(0=Not satisfied; 1=Satisfied; 9=Not known)

16 Inappropriate behaviour

Is the person interfering or objectionable to others?

(exclude specific problems rated under domains 14, 15 & 20)

*Do other people get annoyed, upset or angry because of your behaviour?
What happens?*

CAN1601 CAN1602 CAN1603

Rating	Meaning	Example
0	No need	Such behaviour is not an issue
1	Met need	Under supervision because of potential risk
2	Unmet need	Regular socially unacceptable behaviour
9	Not known	

If rated 0 or 9 go to Question 17

How much help does the person receive from friends or relatives to reduce the risk of disturbing others?

CAN1604 CAN1605 CAN1606

Rating	Meaning	Example
0	None	
1	Low help	Some supervision, weekly or less
2	Moderate help	Supervision several days a week
3	High help	Constant supervision
9	Not known	

How much help does the person *receive* from local services to reduce the risk of disturbing others?

CAN1607 CAN1608 CAN1609

How much help does the person *need* from local services to reduce the risk of disturbing others?

CAN1610 CAN1611 CAN1612

Rating	Meaning	Example
0	None	
1	Low help	Check on behaviour weekly or less, infrequent follow-up
2	Moderate help	Daily supervision. Behaviour management programme
3	High help	Constant supervision, intensive involvement of specialist team, hospitalisations
9	Not known	

Does the person receive the right type of help to reduce the risk of disturbing others?

(0=No; 1=Yes; 9=Not known)

CAN1613 CAN1614 CAN1615

Overall, is the respondent satisfied with the amount of help the person is receiving to reduce the risk of disturbing others?

(0=Not satisfied; 1=Satisfied; 9=Not known)

CAN1616 CAN1617

17 Substance misuse

Does the person have an alcohol or drug problem?

CAN1701 CAN1702 CAN1703

Does drinking alcohol cause you any problems? Do you take any drugs that are not prescribed by the doctor? Do you find it difficult to stop?

Rating	Meaning	Example
0	No need	No alcohol or drug problem
1	Met need	At risk from substance misuse and receiving help
2	Unmet need	Harmful and/or uncontrollable use
9	Not known	

If rated 0 or 9 go to Question 18

How much help does the person receive from friends or relatives for their substance misuse?

CAN1704 CAN1705 CAN1706

Rating	Meaning	Example
0	None	
1	Low help	Occasional advice or support
2	Moderate help	Regular advice, put in touch with helping agencies
3	High help	Daily monitoring of use
9	Not known	

How much help does the person *receive* from local services for their substance misuse?

CAN1707 CAN1708 CAN1709

How much help does the person *need* from local services for their substance misuse?

CAN1710 CAN1711 CAN1712

Rating	Meaning	Example
0	None	
1	Low help	Occasional professional advice
2	Moderate help	Given details of helping agencies. Counselling
3	High help	Attends specialist clinic. Supervised withdrawal programme
9	Not known	

Does the person receive the right type of help for their substance misuse?

CAN1713 CAN1714 CAN1715

(0=No; 1=Yes; 9=Not known)

Overall, is the respondent satisfied with the amount of help the person is receiving for their substance misuse?

CAN1716 CAN1717

(0=Not satisfied; 1=Satisfied; 9=Not known)

18 Communication

Can the person communicate with others?

CAN1801 CAN1802 CAN1803

Can you understand what other people say to you?
Can they understand you?

Rating	Meaning	Example
0	No need	Able to understand and make self understood
1	Met need	Some difficulty, but able to communicate with help
2	Unmet need	Severe problem with understanding or making self understood
9	Not known	

If rated 0 or 9 go to Question 19

How much help does the person receive from friends or relatives for their communication difficulties?

CAN1804 CAN1805 CAN1806

Rating	Meaning	Example
0	None	
1	Low help	Only minimal facilitation of communication
2	Moderate help	Occasional interpretation
3	High help	Accompanies person to make communication possible
9	Not known	

How much help does the person *receive* from local services for their communication difficulties?

CAN1807 CAN1808 CAN1809

How much help does the person *need* from local services for their communication difficulties?

CAN1810 CAN1811 CAN1812

Rating	Meaning	Example
0	None	
1	Low help	Some advice and support
2	Moderate help	Communication skills training
3	High help	Speech therapist involvement
9	Not known	

Does the person receive the right type of help for their communication difficulties?

CAN1813 CAN1814 CAN1815

(0=No; 1=Yes; 9=Not known)

Overall, is the respondent satisfied with the amount of help the person is receiving for their communication difficulties?

CAN1816 CAN1817

(0=Not satisfied; 1=Satisfied; 9=Not known)

19 Social relationships

Assessments

| User rating | Carer rating | Staff rating |

Does the person need help with social contact?

Do you have enough friends? Where do you meet them?
Do you wish you had more contact with other people?

CAN1901 CAN1902 CAN1903

Rating	Meaning	Example
0	No need	Able to organise enough social contact, has enough friends
1	Met need	Needs help with social contact and is receiving it. Attends appropriate drop-in or day centre
2	Unmet need	Frequently feels lonely or isolated
9	Not known	

If rated 0 or 9 go to Question 20

How much help does the person receive from friends or relatives with social contact?

CAN1904 CAN1905 CAN1906

Rating	Meaning	Example
0	None	
1	Low help	Social contact less than weekly
2	Moderate help	Social contact weekly or more often
3	High help	Social contact at least 4 times a week
9	Not known	

How much help does the person *receive* from local services in organising social contact?

CAN1907 CAN1908 CAN1909

How much help does the person *need* from local services in organising social contact?

CAN1910 CAN1911 CAN1912

Rating	Meaning	Example
0	None	
1	Low help	Given advice about social clubs
2	Moderate help	Day centre or comminity group up to 3 times a week
3	High help	Attends day centre 4 or more times a week
9	Not known	

Does the person receive the right type of help in organising social contact?

CAN1913 CAN1914 CAN1915

(0=No; 1=Yes; 9=Not known)

Overall, is the respondent satisfied with the amount of help the person is receiving in organising social contact?

CAN1916 CAN1917

(0=Not satisfied; 1=Satisfied; 9=Not known)

20 Sexual expression

Assessments

| User rating | Carer rating | Staff rating |

Does the person have problems with their sex life?

Do you have any sexual difficulties?

CAN2001 CAN2002 CAN2003

Rating	Meaning	Example
0	No need	Happy with current sex life
1	Met need	Benefiting from sex therapy, sex education programme
2	Unmet need	Serious sexual difficulty. Very limited or no sex life despite existing desire
9	Not known	

If rated 0 or 9 go to Question 21

How much help does the person receive from friends or relatives with problems in their sex life?

CAN2004 CAN2005 CAN2006

Rating	Meaning	Example
0	None	
1	Low help	Some advice
2	Moderate help	Several talks, information material, providing contraceptives
3	High help	Consistent accessibility to talk about the problem. Facilitates contact with counselling services
9	Not known	

How much help does the person *receive* from local services for problems in their sex life?

CAN2007 CAN2008 CAN2009

How much help does the person *need* from local services for problems in their sex life?

CAN2010 CAN2011 CAN2012

Rating	Meaning	Example
0	None	
1	Low help	Some information about sexual matters such as contraception, safe sex, drug-induced impotence
2	Moderate help	Regular discussions on sex issues. Medical investigations
3	High help	Sex therapy. Sex education programme. Other medical/ psychological treatment
9	Not known	

Does the person receive the right type of help for problems in their sex life?

CAN2013 CAN2014 CAN2015

(0=No; 1=Yes; 9=Not known)

Overall, is the respondent satisfied with the amount of help the person is receiving for problems in their sex life?

CAN2016 CAN2017

(0=Not satisfied; 1=Satisfied; 9=Not known)

21 Caring for someone else

Does the person have problems looking after another person?

CAN2101   CAN2102   CAN2103

Do you have any children (under 18) or a relative that you are looking after?
Do you have any difficulty in looking after them?

Rating	Meaning	Example
0	No need	Nobody to look after or no problem with looking after them
1	Met need	Difficulties with caring and receiving help
2	Unmet need	Serious difficulty looking after children or dependent relatives
9	Not known	

If rated 0 or 9 go to Question 22

How much help does the person receive from friends or relatives with looking after children or relatives?

CAN2104   CAN2105   CAN2106

Rating	Meaning	Example
0	None	
1	Low help	Occasional help, less than once a week
2	Moderate help	Help most days of the week
3	High help	Children/sick realtives living with friends or relatives
9	Not known	

How much help does the person *receive* from local services with looking after their children/relatives?

CAN2107   CAN2108   CAN2109

How much help does the person *need* from local services with looking after their children/relatives?

CAN2110   CAN2111   CAN2112

Rating	Meaning	Example
0	None	
1	Low help	Attending day nursery/day care, weekly assistance at home
2	Moderate help	Nearly daily assistance. Given training in caring skills
3	High help	Children/relatives in residential care or other 24-hour care package
9	Not known	

Does the person receive the right type of help for looking after their children/relatives?

CAN2113   CAN2114   CAN2115

(0=No; 1=Yes; 9=Not known)

Overall, is the respondent satisfied with the amount of help the person is receiving with looking after their friends/relatives?

CAN2116   CAN2117

(0=Not satisfied; 1=Satisfied; 9=Not known)

22 Basic education

Does the person lack basic skills in numeracy and literacy?

CAN2201 CAN2202 CAN2203

Do you have difficulty with reading or writing?
Can you count your change in a shop?

Rating	Meaning	Example
0	No need	Able to read, write and understand English
1	Met need	Difficulty with reading and has help
2	Unmet need	Serious difficulties with basic skills
9	Not known	

If rated 0 or 9 go to Question 23

How much help does the person receive from friends or relatives with numeracy and literacy?

CAN2204 CAN2205 CAN2206

Rating	Meaning	Example
0	None	
1	Low help	Occasional help to read or fill in forms
2	Moderate help	Has put them in touch with literacy classes
3	High help	Teaches the person to read
9	Not known	

How much help does the person *receive* from local services with numeracy and literacy?

CAN2207 CAN2208 CAN2209

How much help does the person *need* from local services with numeracy and literacy?

CAN2210 CAN2211 CAN2212

Rating	Meaning	Example
0	None	
1	Low help	Help filling in forms
2	Moderate help	Given advice about classes
3	High help	Attending adult education
9	Not known	

Does the person receive the right type of help with numeracy and literacy?

CAN2213 CAN2214 CAN2215

(0=No; 1=Yes; 9=Not known)

Overall, is the respondent satisfied with the amount of help the person is receiving with numeracy and literacy?

CAN2216 CAN2217

(0=Not satisfied; 1=Satisfied; 9=Not known)

23 Transport

Does the person have any problems using public transport?

CAN2301 CAN2302 CAN2303

How do you go to different places outside your house? Can you travel by bus, tube or train? Does anyone help you? Do you have a free bus pass?

Rating	Meaning	Example
0	No need	Able to use public transport, or has access to car
1	Met need	Bus pass or other help provided with transport
2	Unmet need	Unable to use public transport. No other transport easily available
9	Not known	

If rated 0 or 9 go to Question 24

How much help does the person receive from friends or relatives with travelling?

CAN2304 CAN2305 CAN2306

Rating	Meaning	Example
0	None	
1	Low help	Encouragement to travel
2	Moderate help	Often accompanies on public transport
3	High help	Provides transport to all appointments
9	Not known	

How much help does the person *receive* from local services with travelling?

CAN2307 CAN2308 CAN2309

How much help does the person *need* from local services with travelling?

CAN2310 CAN2311 CAN2312

Rating	Meaning	Example
0	None	
1	Low help	Provision of bus pass
2	Moderate help	Taxi card
3	High help	Transport to appointments by ambulance, etc.
9	Not known	

Does the person receive the right type of help with travelling?

CAN2313 CAN2314 CAN2315

(0=No; 1=Yes; 9=Not known)

Overall, is the respondent satisfied with the amount of help the person is receiving with travelling?

CAN2316 CAN2317

(0=Not satisfied; 1=Satisfied; 9=Not known)

24 Money budgeting

Does the person have problems budgeting their money?

How do you find budgeting your money?
Do you manage to pay your bills yourself? Does anyone help you?

CAN2401 CAN2402 CAN2403

Rating	Meaning	Example
0	No need	Able to buy essential items and pay bills
1	Met need	Benefits from help with budgeting
2	Unmet need	Unable to manage finances
9	Not known	

If rated 0 or 9 go to Question 25

How much help does the person receive from friends or relatives in managing their money?

CAN2404 CAN2405 CAN2406

Rating	Meaning	Example
0	None	
1	Low help	Occasional help sorting out household bills
2	Moderate help	Calculating weekly budget
3	High help	Complete control of finances
9	Not known	

How much help does the person *receive* from local services in managing their money?

CAN2407 CAN2408 CAN2409

How much help does the person *need* from local services in managing their money?

CAN2410 CAN2411 CAN2412

Rating	Meaning	Example
0	None	
1	Low help	Occasional help with budgeting
2	Moderate help	Supervised in paying rent, given weekly spending money
3	High help	Daily handouts of cash
9	Not known	

Does the person receive the right type of help in managing their money?

CAN2413 CAN2414 CAN2415

(0=No; 1=Yes; 9=Not known)

Overall, is the respondent satisfied with the amount of help the person is receiving in managing their money?

CAN2416 CAN2417

(0=Not satisfied; 1=Satisfied; 9=Not known)

25 Welfare benefits

Assessments

User rating | Carer rating | Staff rating

Is the person definitely receiving all the benefits that they are entitled to?

CAN2501 CAN2502 CAN2503

Are you sure that you are getting all the benefits you are entitled to?

Rating	Meaning	Example
0	No need	Receiving full entitlement of benefits
1	Met need	Receives appropriate help in claiming benefits
2	Unmet need	Not sure/not receiving full entitlement of benefits
9	Not known	

If rated 0 or 9 CANDID–R is completed

How much help does the person receive from friends or relatives in obtaining their full benefit entitlement?

CAN2504 CAN2505 CAN2506

Rating	Meaning	Example
0	None	
1	Low help	Occasionally asks whether person is getting any money
2	Moderate help	Has helped fill in forms
3	High help	Has made enquiries about full entitlement
9	Not known	

How much help does the person *receive* from local services in obtaining their full benefit entitlement?

CAN2507 CAN2508 CAN2509

How much help does the person *need* from local services in obtaining their full benefit entitlement?

CAN2510 CAN2511 CAN2512

Rating	Meaning	Example
0	None	
1	Low help	Occasional advice about entitlements
2	Moderate help	Help with applying for extra entitlements
3	High help	Comprehensive evaluation of current entitlement
9	Not known	

Does the person receive the right type of help in obtaining their full benefit entitlement?

CAN2513 CAN2514 CAN2515

(0=No; 1=Yes; 9=Not known)

Overall, is the respondent satisfied with the amount of help the person is receiving for obtaining their full benefit entitlement?

CAN2516 CAN2517

(0=Not satisfied; 1=Satisfied; 9=Not known)

Appendix 3

CANDID–R rating sheets

Suggested rating sheets for CANDID–R

User, carer and staff rating sheets

These score sheets summarise the data collected during a CANDID–R interview, giving a condensed record of the full interview. In addition, they provide space for recording the summary scores. Separate sheets are available for user, carer and staff assessments.

CANDID–S is a self-contained document, and so does not need a separate summary sheet.

CANDID–R
User rating sheet

User name _____ Date of assessment _____/_____/_____

Interviewer's name _____

	Section 1 need identified	Section 2 informal help given	Section 3 formal help given/needed		Section 4 satisfaction type/amount	
Rating (9 = not known)	0, 1 or 2	0, 1, 2 or 3	0, 1, 2 or 3		0 or 1	
CANDID box number	01	04	07	10	13	16
1 Accommodation						
2 Food						
3 Looking after the home						
4 Self-care						
5 Daytime activities						
6 General physical health						
7 Eyesight/hearing						
8 Mobility						
9 Seizures						
10 Major mental health problems						
11 Other mental health problems						
12 Information						
13 Exploitation risk						
14 Safety of self						
15 Safety of others						
16 Inappropriate behaviour						
17 Substance misuse						
18 Communication						
19 Social relationships						
20 Sexual expression						
21 Caring for someone else						
22 Basic education						
23 Transport						
24 Money budgeting						
25 Welfare benefits						
Number of met needs (Number of 1s)						
Number of unmet needs (Number of 2s)						
Total number of needs (Number of 1s and 2s)						
Total level of help given & needed (Add scores, rate 9 as 0)						

CANDID–R
Carer rating sheet

User name _____ Date of assessment _____/_____/_____

Interviewer's name _____

Carer's name and relationship _____

	Section 1 need identified	Section 2 informal help given	Section 3 formal help given/needed		Section 4 satisfaction type/amount	
Rating (9 = not known)	0, 1 or 2	0, 1, 2 or 3	0, 1, 2 or 3		0 or 1	
CANDID box number	02	05	08	11	14	17
1 Accommodation						
2 Food						
3 Looking after the home						
4 Self-care						
5 Daytime activities						
6 General physical health						
7 Eyesight/hearing						
8 Mobility						
9 Seizures						
10 Major mental health problems						
11 Other mental health problems						
12 Information						
13 Exploitation risk						
14 Sefety of self						
15 Safety of others						
16 Inappropriate behaviour						
17 Substance misuse						
18 Communication						
19 Social relationships						
20 Sexual expression						
21 Caring for someone else						
22 Basic education						
23 Transport						
24 Money budgeting						
25 Welfare benefits						
Number of met needs (Number of 1s)						
Number of unmet needs (Number of 2s)						
Total number of needs (Number of 1s and 2s)						
Total level of help given & needed (Add scores, rate 9 as 0)						

CANDID–R
Staff rating sheet

User name _____ Date of assessment ____/____/____

Interviewer's name _____

Staff name and designation _____

	Section 1 need identified	**Section 2** informal help given	**Section 3** formal help given/needed		**Section 4** satisfaction type/amount	
Rating (9 = not known)	0, 1 or 2	0, 1, 2 or 3	0, 1, 2 or 3		0 or 1	
CANDID box number	03	06	09	12	15	
1 Accommodation						
2 Food						
3 Looking after the home						
4 Self-care						
5 Daytime activities						
6 General physical health						
7 Eyesight/hearing						
8 Mobility						
9 Seizures						
10 Major mental health problems						
11 Other mental health problems						
12 Information						
13 Exploitation risk						
14 Sefety of self						
15 Safety of others						
16 Inappropriate behaviour						
17 Substance misuse						
18 Communication						
19 Social relationships						
20 Sexual expression						
21 Caring for someone else						
22 Basic education						
23 Transport						
24 Money budgeting						
25 Welfare benefits						
Number of met needs (Number of 1s)						
Number of unmet needs (Number of 2s)						
Total number of needs (Number of 1s and 2s)						
Total level of help given & needed (Add scores, rate 9 as 0)						

Appendix 4

Training overheads

1 Needs assessment in learning disabilities

- Definition of need & importance of needs assessment

- Services should be provided on the basis of need

- Everyone has needs arising from a variety of causes

- Needs can be met or unmet

- The views of staff about need can differ from those of service users and their carers

2 CANDID: introduction

- Known and acceptable validity and reliability

- Brief and suitable for use by a range of professionals

- Requires no formal training

- Records the points of view of the service user, informal carer and staff

- Measures met and unmet need

- Measures the help provided by informal carers and services separately

- Suitable for research and clinical use

3 CANDID: need domains

1   Accommodation
2   Food
3   Looking after the home
4   Self-care
5   Daytime activities
6   General physical health
7   Eyesight/hearing
8   Mobility
9   Seizures
10 Major mental health problems
11 Other mental health problems
12 Information
13 Exploitation risk
14 Safety of self
15 Safety of others
16 Inappropriate behaviour
17 Substance misuse
18 Communication
19 Social relationships
20 Sexual expression
21 Caring for someone else
22 Basic education
23 Transport
24 Money budgeting
25 Welfare benefits

4a CANDID–R
SAFETY OF OTHERS ASSESSMENT PAGE (Sections 1 & 2)

Assessments

	User rating	Carer rating	Staff rating

Is the person a current or potential risk to other peoples' safety?

Do you think you could be a danger to other people?
Do you ever lose your temper and hit people?

Rating	Meaning	Example
0	No need	No history of violence or threatening behaviour
1	Met need	Under supervision because of potential risk
2	Unmet need	Recent violence or threats
9	Not known	

If rated 0 or 9 go to Question 16

CAN1501   CAN1502   CAN1503

How much help does the person receive from friends or relatives to reduce the risk that they might harm someone else?

Rating	Meaning	Example
0	None	
1	Low help	Help with threatening behaviour weekly or less
2	Moderate help	Help with threatening behaviour more than weekly
3	High help	Almost constant help with persistently threatening behaviour
9	Not known	

CAN1504   CAN1505   CAN1506

4b CANDID–R
SAFETY OF OTHERS ASSESSMENT PAGE (Sections 3 & 4)

How much help does the person *receive* from local services to reduce the risk that they might harm someone else?

CAN1507 CAN1508 CAN1509

How much help does the person *need* from local services to reduce the risk that they might harm someone else?

CAN1510 CAN1511 CAN1512

Rating	Meaning	Example
0	None	
1	Low help	Check on behaviour weekly or less
2	Moderate help	Daily supervision
3	High help	Constant supervision, anger management programme
9	Not known	

Does the person receive the right type of help to reduce the risk that they might harm someone else?

CAN1513 CAN1514 CAN1515

(0=No; 1=Yes; 9=Not known)

Overall, is the respondent satisfied with the amount of help the person is receiving to reduce the risk that they might harm someone else?

CAN1516 CAN1517

(0=Not satisfied; 1=Satisfied; 9=Not known)

5 Met and unmet need (CANDID–R Section 1 or CANDID–S)

- A need is met if the person has no problem or a moderate problem in the domain, due to the help given (rating 1)

- A need is unmet if the person has a current serious problem in the domain, irrespective of help given (rating 2)

- There is no need if the person has no problem in the domain and no help is given (rating 0)

- The rating is not known if the person does not know or does not wish to answer (rating 9)

6 Help and satisfaction (CANDID–R Sections 2, 3 & 4)

- Section 2 assesses informal help given

- Section 3a assesses formal help given

- Section 3b assesses formal help needed

- Rating key identical for Sections 2 & 3
    - 0=no help
    - 1=low help
    - 2=moderate help
    - 3=high help
    - 9=not known

- Section 4a assesses satisfaction with type and 4b amount of help

- Rating: 0=not satisfied; 1=satisfied; 9=not known

Appendix 5

Training vignettes

(a) Brief practice vignette with ratings in the *Safety of others* domain.
(b) Full vignette with completed CANDID–R rating sheets.

Brief practice vignette

The goal is to have a first attempt at rating the CANDID. The domain 'Safety of others' was chosen as a typical domain for practice. The expected ratings are given so that the procedure to arrive at these ratings can be discussed in the training session. For CANDID–S training, only the ratings for Section 1 are required.

Interview with John – a service user

John is a 31-year-old man with moderate learning disabilities who lives in a supported group home, but his current community placement is in jeopardy because of his aggressive behaviour. For the past 6 months he has been pushing, hitting and throwing cups at other service users and staff. He has been prescribed some sedative medication by his general practitioner but it has not helped much. The home staff had to increase their level of support and provide one-to-one attention for long periods every day. His mother visits him almost every day and this seems to calm him down. Staff at the home think John should be admitted to the psychiatric ward because they are no longer able to manage his behaviour safely. His mother thinks that 'he is not that bad', home staff are 'excellent' and that between them and herself (mother) John's behaviour is currently under control. John does not admit to hitting anybody, nor does he agree that he needs help with controlling his temper.

Rating of practice vignette in the *Safety of others* domain

Section 1 (need rating)

User rating	0 (no need)
Carer rating	1 (met need)
Staff rating	2 (unmet need)

Section 2 (informal help)

User rating	no rating
Carer rating	2 (moderate help)
Staff rating	2 (moderate help)

Section 3 (formal help)

User rating	no rating
Carer rating	a) 2 (moderate help received)
	b) 2 (moderate help needed)
Staff rating	a) 2 (moderate help received)
	b) 3 (high help needed)

Section 4 (satisfaction)

User rating	no rating
Carer rating	a) 1 (satisfied with type of help)
	b) 1 (satisfied with amount of help)
Staff rating	a) 0 (not satisfied with type of help)
	b) no rating

Full vignette

Michelle's needs assessment is given here from three different perspectives. Information from the interviews with Michelle (user), her father (informal carer) and her social worker (staff) are provided, followed by CANDID–R rating sheets completed on the basis of these interviews. For CANDID–S training, only the ratings for Section 1 are required and CANDID–S (Appendix 1) sheets are used for recording.

Interview with Michelle X

Michelle lives in a 24-hour supported staff home for people with mild learning disabilities and mental health problems, and she likes it there. Her social worker arranged for her to move there 2 months ago. She enjoys cooking and is able to cook her own meals, occasionally cooking for the other two residents as well. However, she needs some help both with shopping and in the kitchen. Although she admits that she is not the tidiest person, she does not need any reminding to keep her room and herself clean. She attends a day centre 4 days a week and she enjoys that. Her father visits her usually a couple of evenings a week, and they go out for a walk or a coffee. She suffers from diabetes, for which she attends the Diabetes Clinic at the local hospital on her own and takes tablets regularly. She is fully mobile and has no hearing or eyesight problems. She had epileptic fits as a child but not since for many years, and she is on no anti-epileptic medication.

She knows that she has manic depression and feels that taking lithium has helped her. She sees her psychiatrist every 4–5 months and she thinks that's fine. Michelle knows a lot about her illness and lithium because her community psychiatric nurse (CPN), whom she is currently seeing once a month, explains it all to her. Although she has harmed herself in the past when she was feeling depressed, she has had no self-harm thoughts recently. She attributes this to her medication and the support she is getting from her CPN. She has hit her care workers in the past, but this was because they were 'winding her up'. She does not feel like hitting anyone currently and this is not because of any help she is receiving – she said 'I'm just not a violent person'. She does not think that her behaviour is ever annoying or embarrassing to other people.

She has several friends that she meets regularly at the day centre and she enjoys her father's company. She does not have a sex life, but she does not see this as a problem as she does not want to have a sexual relationship. She feels she can stand up for herself and is not at risk of being taken advantage of. She has a mild speech impediment but says that people can understand her with no problem; however, at interview it was quite difficult to understand her speech. She had some speech therapy several years ago that she thinks has helped a lot. She can read and write and she does not have anyone else to care for. She does not drink or take illicit drugs. She has a bus pass and can travel independently within a certain range from her home. She has no difficulty budgeting and has a social worker, who is sorting out her benefits for her, and she knows that she gets all the benefits she is entitled to.

Interview with Michelle's father

Mr X felt that Michelle's current accommodation is the right place for her and was very pleased that she moved from her previous placement. He said that she is very good with cooking but she needs some help and supervision. She needs to be prompted to wash herself, and staff have to clean her room regularly because she would not do it. He thinks that the day centre is very helpful in terms of both daytime activities and socialising, but he does not think it needs to be as frequent as it is now. He does not provide any help with her home or self care because staff do this. She has a diagnosis of manic depression for which she is on lithium, but she has been fine mood-wise in the past month. He thinks that her mental health is stable now, as a result of this care. He does not think that the CPN does or needs to explain to her about her illness because he reads a lot about mental health issues himself, tries to support Michelle and provides her with useful leaflets, so he believes she is well informed. He is concerned about her angry outbursts, as they can be quite bad (throwing things at people, shouting and screaming, swearing, etc.) and he thinks that she would benefit from seeing a psychologist, which is not currently happening. He was very worried when she used to cut her wrists, but feels that her CPN and psychiatrist are helping her a lot in that respect and her own safety is not a problem now. He feels that she is protected in her current environment but that she would be open to exploitation if it were not for the support she is getting from home staff. He also thinks that she would benefit from sexual counselling, as she knows nothing about these things. She does not abuse drugs or alcohol. People have difficulty understanding her because of her speech impediment – he sees this as a serious problem and is concerned that nothing is being done about it. She does not have any relatives she looks after. She can budget her money relatively well but only if she is given occasional guidance, which both staff and Mr X provide. He is not sure if she gets all the money she is entitled to.

Interview with Michelle's social worker

He is pleased that Michelle now has a new home, as he believes that her previous placement was totally inappropriate. He knows that she likes cooking, but he thinks that she needs a lot of help with shopping and preparing meals, which is given by home staff. He believes that she would have a serious problem with both her self-care and looking after her room if it were not for care staff prompting her. He has arranged for her to attend the day centre and believes that this is exactly what she needs to be meaningfully occupied during the day. He is aware of her history of epilepsy and diabetes, but is not sure about what medical follow-up she is receiving. He does not believe that she needs any help with her mobility, hearing or eyesight. Her mood swings used to be really bad but he thinks that she is well maintained on her current medication regime. He thinks that her CPN is doing a good job with keeping her informed about her manic depression and lithium treatment and he knows that her father is interested in mental health issues and regularly provides her with magazines, newsletters, etc. He acknowledges that her behaviour in terms of aggression to others has been a serious problem in the past, but not at all recently, which he thinks is primarily because of good compliance with lithium, CPN follow-up and out-patient appointments. For the same reason, her self-harm is not a problem currently. He has arranged a number of social activities for her, and her father regularly spends time with her. He believes that without these arrangements she would be isolated and lonely. He knows that her sex life is non-existent and she does not mind this, but he feels that this is because she is scared to start a sexual relationship due to her very poor sexual knowledge. So he thinks that she could be helped by sex education, which she has never had. In terms of communication, he knows that her comprehension is very good but that people have great difficulty understanding her. He does not know, however, what can be done to alleviate this problem, as speech therapy some years ago did not seem to help. She needs no help with reading or writing and can travel independently using her bus pass. He knows that she is getting all the benefits that she is entitled to, but that she needs a bit of help with money budgeting, which she is currently getting from staff and her father.

CANDID–R
User rating sheet

User name Michelle   Date of assessment   19   /   05   /   03

Interviewer's name Jane D (CPN)

	Section 1 need identified	Section 2 informal help given	Section 3 formal help given/needed		Section 4 satisfaction type/amount	
Rating (9 = not known)	0, 1 or 2	0, 1, 2 or 3	0, 1, 2 or 3		0 or 1	
CANDID box number	01	04	07	10	13	16
1 Accommodation	1	0	3	3	1	1
2 Food	1	0	1	1	1	1
3 Looking after the home	0					
4 Self-care	0					
5 Daytime activities	1	0	2	2	1	1
6 General physical health	1	0	2	2	1	1
7 Eyesight/hearing	0					
8 Mobility	0					
9 Seizures	0					
10 Major mental health problems	1	0	1	1	1	1
11 Other mental health problems	0					
12 Information	1	0	1	1	1	1
13 Exploitation risk	0					
14 Safety of self	1	0	1	1	1	1
15 Safety of others	0					
16 Inappropriate behaviour	0					
17 Substance misuse	0					
18 Communication	0					
19 Social relations	1	2	2	2	1	1
20 Sexual expression	0					
21 Caring for someone else	0					
22 Basic education	0					
23 Transport	1	0	1	1	1	1
24 Money budgeting	0					
25 Welfare benefits	1					
Number of met needs (Number of 1s)	10					
Number of unmet needs (Number of 2s)	0					
Total number of needs (Number of 1s and 2s)	10					
Total level of help given & needed (Add scores, rate 9 as 0)		2	14	14	9	9

CANDID–R
Carer rating sheet

User name Michelle X _____ Date of assessment 20 / 05 / 03

Interviewer's name Jane D (CPN) _____

Carer's name and relationship Mr X (father) _____

	Section 1 need identified	Section 2 informal help given	Section 3 formal help given/needed		Section 4 satisfaction type/amount	
Rating (9 = not known)	0, 1 or 2	0, 1, 2 or 3	0, 1, 2 or 3		0 or 1	
CANDID box number	02	05	08	11	14	17
1 Accommodation	1	0	3	3	1	1
2 Food	1	0	1	1	1	1
3 Looking after the home	1	0	2	2	1	1
4 Self-care	1	0	1	1	1	1
5 Daytime activities	1	0	2	2	1	1
6 General physical health	1	0	2	2	1	1
7 Eyesight/hearing	0					
8 Mobility	0					
9 Seizures	0					
10 Major mental health problems	1	1	1	1	1	1
11 Other mental health problems	0					
12 Information	1	1	0	0	1	1
13 Exploitation risk	1	0	1	1	1	1
14 Safety of self	1	0	1	1	1	1
15 Safety of others	2	0	0	2	0	0
16 Inappropriate behaviour	0					
17 Substance misuse	0					
18 Communication	2	0	0	1	0	0
19 Social relations	1	2	2	2	1	1
20 Sexual expression	2	0	0	2	0	0
21 Caring for someone else	0					
22 Basic education	0					
23 Transport	1	0	1	1	1	1
24 Money budgeting	1	1	1	1	1	1
25 Welfare benefits	9					
Number of met needs (Number of 1s)	13					
Number of unmet needs (Number of 2s)	3					
Total number of needs (Number of 1s and 2s)	16					
Total level of help given & needed (Add scores, rate 9 as 0)		5	18	23	13	13

CANDID–R
Staff rating sheet

User name Michelle X   Date of assessment   20 / 05 / 03

Interviewer's name Jane D (CPN)

Staff name and designation George C (social worker)

	Section 1 need identified	Section 2 informal help given	Section 3 formal help given/needed		Section 4 satisfaction type/amount	
Rating (9 = not known)	0, 1 or 2	0, 1, 2 or 3	0, 1, 2 or 3		0 or 1	
CANDID box number	03	06	09	12	15	
1 Accommodation	1	0	3	3	1	
2 Food	1	0	2	2	1	
3 Looking after the home	1	0	1	1	1	
4 Self-care	1	0	1	1	1	
5 Daytime activities	1	0	2	2	1	
6 General physical health	9					
7 Eyesight/hearing	0					
8 Mobility	0					
9 Seizures	0					
10 Major mental health problems	1	9	1	1	1	
11 Other mental health problems	0					
12 Information	1	1	1	1	1	
13 Exploitation risk	1	0	1	1	1	
14 Safety of self	1	0	1	1	1	
15 Safety of others	1	0	1	1	1	
16 Inappropriate behaviour	0					
17 Substance misuse	0					
18 Communication	2	0	0	3	0	
19 Social relations	1	2	2	2	1	
20 Sexual expression	2	0	0	1	1	
21 Caring for someone else	0					
22 Basic education	0					
23 Transport	1	0	1	1	1	
24 Money budgeting	1	1	1	1	1	
25 Welfare benefits	1	0	3	3	1	
Number of met needs (Number of 1s)	14					
Number of unmet needs (Number of 2s)	2					
Total number of needs (Number of 1s and 2s)	16					
Total level of help given & needed (Add scores, rate 9 as 0)		4	21	25	15	

© *The Royal College of Psychiatrists, 2003. This page may be photocopied freely.*

Appendix 6

CANDID reliability and validity

Reprinted from the *British Journal of Psychiatry* (2000), vol. 176, pp. 473–478; incorporating corrigendum published (2000), vol. 177, p. 184.

BRITISH JOURNAL OF PSYCHIATRY (2000), 176, 473–478

Reliability and validity of the CANDID – a needs assessment instrument for adults with learning disabilities and mental health problems

K. XENITIDIS, G. THORNICROFT, M. LEESE, M. SLADE, M. FOTIADOU,
H. PHILP, J. SAYER, E. HARRIS, D. McGEE and D. G. M. MURPHY

Background People with learning disabilities and mental health problems have complex needs. Care should be provided according to need.

Aim To develop a standardised needs-assessment instrument for adults with learning disabilities and mental health problems.

Method The Camberwell Assessment of Need for Adults with Developmental and Intellectual Disabilities (CANDID) was developed by modifying the Camberwell Assessment of Need (CAN). Concurrent validity was tested using the Global Assessment of Functioning (GAF) and the Disability Assessment Schedule (DAS). Test–retest and interrater reliability were investigated using 40 adults with learning disabilities and mental health problems.

Results CANDID scores were significantly correlated with both DAS ($P < 0.05$) and GAF scores ($P < 0.01$). Correlation coefficients for interrater reliability were 0.93 (user), 0.90 (carer), and 0.97 (staff ratings); for test–retest reliability they were 0.71, 0.69 and 0.86 respectively. Mean interview duration was less than 30 minutes.

Conclusions The CANDID is a brief, valid and reliable needs assessment instrument for adults with learning disabilities and mental health problems.

Declaration of interest K.X. was supported by the National Health Service Executive (South Thames).

Following the closure of mental handicap hospitals, most adults with learning disabilities receive care in various community settings at a substantial cost. The National Health Service (NHS) and local authorities spend approximately £1 000 000 000 on services for people with learning disabilities (Audit Commission, 1992). The *NHS and Community Care Act* (House of Commons, 1990) established a statutory duty on social services to assess the needs of people who may require community care. The Camberwell Assessment of Need (CAN; Phelan *et al*, 1995) is an established needs-assessment instrument for those with severe mental illness. Although people with learning disabilities are more likely to develop mental health problems than their non-disabled counterparts (Reiss, 1994), there is no widely accepted instrument for measuring needs in this group. This study aimed to develop the Camberwell Assessment of Need for Adults with Developmental and Intellectual Disabilities (CANDID) and investigate its validity and reliability.

METHOD

Development of the CANDID

The CANDID was developed by modifying the CAN to make its content relevant to adults with learning disabilities and mental health problems while retaining its format and structure. The CANDID shares with the CAN the criteria set prior to the latter's development, namely that it should:

(a) have acceptable validity and reliability;

(b) be brief and suitable for use by a range of professionals;

(c) require no formal training;

(d) record separately the views of the service users, their informal carers and staff;

(e) measure met and unmet need;

(f) assess the help provided by informal carers and local services;

(g) be suitable for clinical and research use.

The questions in each of the 25 need areas of the CANDID are divided into four sections: Section 1 assesses the absence or presence of need, and, if present, whether it is met or unmet; Section 2 rates the help received from informal carers; Section 3 asks how much help by local services is provided (3a) and needed (3b); Section 4 inquires about the respondent's satisfaction with the type (4a) and amount (4b) of help received from local services.

First draft

Focus groups of service users, informal carers and staff identified areas of needs relevant to people with learning disabilities and mental health problems. The users group ($n=8$) consisted of adults with mild or moderate learning disabilities who were attending a day centre or were living in local residential facilities. The carers group ($n=7$) consisted of informal carers of people using the above facilities. The staff group ($n=9$) consisted of staff from a variety of disciplines working with people with learning disabilities and mental health problems. The first draft of the instrument was developed using findings from these focus groups.

Second draft

The first draft was commented on by health and social services professionals ($n=24$) with expertise in working with adults with learning disabilities and mental health problems. These consultations were conducted on an individual basis and focused on the content and structure of the instrument and its usefulness in research and clinical settings. Case vignettes were used, taking into account the whole range of the target population. As a result of these consultations the second draft was developed.

Validity studies

Content validity

We designed a questionnaire that asked about the views of service users ($n=45$) and their informal carers on the list of need areas identified through the process described above. Users and carers were asked to score each need area item according to its relevance, and to suggest any additional items that should have been included. Adults with all levels of learning disabilities were included in this sample. For those with a level of learning disability severe enough to interfere significantly with the comprehension of the questionnaire, it was completed by carers alone.

Consensual validity

Fifty-five experts in the field of mental health in people with learning disabilities from a range of professional backgrounds and all parts of the UK were surveyed. Their opinion was sought on the content, language and structure of the CANDID by mailing them a copy of the second draft accompanied by a questionnaire inviting them to rate, on a five-point Likert scale, 'helpfulness of anchor points', 'ease of use' and 'appropriateness of language'.

Criterion validity

No 'gold standard' needs-assessment instrument currently exists for people with learning disabilities and mental health problems. In order to establish the concurrent validity of the CANDID, two instruments were used: the Disability Assessment Schedule (DAS; Holmes et al, 1982); and the Global Assessment of Functioning (GAF; American Psychiatric Association, 1994). The DAS was developed in order to assess level of functioning in 12 life areas of people with learning disabilities; the GAF measures global level of psychiatric symptom severity and disability. Concurrent validity was calculated in two ways: first CANDID summary scores (total number of needs) rated by staff were compared with total DAS and GAF scores; second, a comparison was made between DAS scores in individual areas of need (behaviour, communication, mobility, social interaction and self-care) and corresponding areas of the CANDID. These areas were selected because they were the overlapping areas in the two instruments that could be meaningfully compared.

Predictive validity is relative to a needs-assessment instrument because of its capacity to predict future service utilisation and therefore assist with needs-led service planning. However, no attempt was made to establish the predictive validity of the CANDID because this would require a longitudinal study design, which was beyond the scope of this study.

Reliability studies

Sample acquisition

Two sampling frames were used: first, all adults (n=210) using a community-based specialist learning disabilities mental health service in an outer London borough (Bromley); second, all in-patients (n=12) of a national unit for adults with mild or moderate learning disabilities at a psychiatric hospital (Bethlem Royal Hospital). The community subsample (n=31), although not randomly selected, included people with a range of levels of intellectual ability and a variety of mental health and behavioural problems characteristic of users of specialist learning disability mental health services. The in-patient subsample comprised nine people, after three patients were judged by their consultant psychiatrist to be too disturbed to participate. Thus, 40 people in total were recruited for the reliability study. Only one of those approached refused to participate. An estimate based on the original CAN data had indicated that for interrater reliability a sample of this size would be adequate to estimate an intraclass correlation of 0.88 to within ±0.1 with approximately 95% confidence.

Reliability study design

Five interviewer/raters were used: a psychiatrist, an occupational therapist, a social worker and two nurses. A brief explanation of the scope of the instrument and the rating procedure, but no formal training, was given.

Forty subject trios, each consisting of a service user, their informal carer and a member of staff, were enrolled in the reliability study. Of these, nine users could not be interviewed owing to the severity of their learning disabilities, and 13 carers were unavailable. Hence for the investigation of interrater reliability, 31 users, 27 carers and 40 staff were interviewed at a given point of time (T_1). All interviews performed at T_1 were timed. With 29 of the 40 triplets the interviews were conducted 'live' by an interviewer in the presence of a silent second rater (all five raters rotated in their role as interviewer or second rater). The remaining 11 trios were interviewed by one interviewer alone (the same interviewer conducting all interviews), and the interviews were audio-taped. All four second raters rated the taped material at a later stage.

For the test–retest reliability exercise, the same interviewer who performed interviews at T_1 re-interviewed the respondents at a second point in time (T_2), this time alone. The interval between T_1 and T_2 was on average 11 days, and 77.5% of the subjects were re-interviewed at T_2. For the taped interviews (where all four second raters rated the same material), reliability was estimated separately for each second rater, and the overall reliability was calculated.

Statistical analysis

For testing criterion validity, non-parametric correlation (Spearman's r) and Student's t-test were used. Interrater and test–retest reliability were examined for the total number of needs and for each need item individually. For the reliability of individual items, two measures of agreement were calculated: complete percentage agreement and unweighted k coefficient. For the reliability of the total number of needs, variance component estimation was performed using the MINQUE (minimum norm quadratic unbiased estimation) method in the Statistical Package for the Social Sciences (SPSS) version 7.5 for Windows (SPSS, 1996). Variance components estimation is a flexible method of obtaining reliability coefficients if there are several sources of variation, and the MINQUE method is robust concerning moderate departure from normality (Dunn, 1992). For interrater estimates, both patient variation and rater variation were estimated as random effects. For test–retest estimates, time was included as a fixed effect. Each interclass correlation coefficient was estimated as the ratio of variation between subjects to total variation. Relative bias in T_2 estimates compared with T_1 estimates was tested by using a paired t-test. Fixed effects between raters were tested by using a fixed effect analysis of variance. Also, a Student's t-test was used to compare the mean differences in the ratings of users, carers and staff for the comparison of the individual DAS scores in the two CANDID groups.

RESULTS

Socio-demographic characteristics and needs profile of the study sample

The characteristics of the 40 service users recruited for the reliability study are shown in Table 1.

The mean total number of needs per user identified at T_1 by the users themselves (n=31) was 11.55 (s.d.=2.51, 95% CI 10.63–12.47), while informal carers (n=27) identified 14.10 needs (s.d.=2.34, 95% CI 13.11–14.96) and staff (n=40) identified 13.98 (s.d.=2.97, 95% CI 13.03–14.92). The ratings by carers and staff did not differ significantly, whereas the ratings by

Table 1 Characteristics of patients enrolled in the reliability study (*n*=40)

Characteristic	Value
Age (years; mean (range))	37.5 (20–67)
Gender (*n* (%))	
Male	27 (67.5%)
Female	13 (32.5%)
Ethnic origin (*n* (%))	
Caucasian	38 (95%)
African–Caribbean	1 (2.5%)
Asian	1 (2.5%)
Patient status (*n* (%))	
Outpatient	15 (37.5%)
Inpatient	9 (2.5%)
Residential	16 (40%)
Level of learning disability (*n* (%))	
Mild	26 (65%)
Moderate	19 (22.5%)
Severe/profound	5 (12.5%)
Living situation (*n* (%))	
Alone	2 (5%)
With partner	2 (5%)
With parents	9 (22.5%)
With others	27 (67.5%)
Marital status (*n* (%))	
Single	37 (92.5%)
Married	3 (7.5%)
Clinical conditions (*n* (%))	
Psychotic illness	20 (50%)
Autism	10 (25%)
Epilepsy	11 (27.5%)

Table 2 Assessment of need for the 25 areas of the CANDID

Area of need	No serious need (n (%))	Met need (n (%))	Unmet need (n (%))	Not known (n (%))
Accommodation	0 (0)	36 (90)	4 (10)	0 (0)
Food	1 (2.5)	38 (95)	0 (0)	1 (2.5)
Looking after the home	6 (15)	30 (75)	2 (5)	2 (5)
Self-care	6 (15)	33 (82.5)	0 (0)	1 (2.5)
Daytime activities	3 (7.5)	33 (82.5)	4 (10)	0 (0)
General physical health	22 (55)	18 (45)	0 (0)	0 (0)
Eyesight and hearing	24 (60)	16 (40)	0 (0)	0 (0)
Mobility	35 (87.5)	5 (12.5)	0 (0)	0 (0)
Seizures	32 (80)	7 (17.5)	1 (2.5)	0 (0)
Major mental health problems	21 (52.5)	16 (40)	3 (7.5)	0 (0)
Minor mental health problems	6 (15)	28 (70)	6 (15)	0 (0)
Information	28 (70)	8 (20)	0 (0)	4 (10)
Safety to self	21 (52.5)	17 (42.5)	2 (5)	0 (0)
Exploitation risk	11 (27.5)	27 (67.5)	2 (5)	0 (0)
Safety to others	18 (45)	14 (35)	8 (20)	0 (0)
Inappropriate behaviour	20 (50)	16 (40)	4 (10)	0 (0)
Substance misuse	37 (92.5)	3 (7.5)	0 (0)	0 (0)
Communication	20 (50)	18 (45)	2 (5)	0 (0)
Social relationship	6 (15)	26 (65)	7 (17.5)	0 (0)
Sexual expression	25 (62.5)	10 (25)	4 (10)	1 (2.5)
Caring for someone else	37 (92.5)	1 (2.5)	2 (5)	0 (0)
Basic education	3 (7.5)	27 (67.5)	8 (20)	2 (5)
Transport	6 (15)	28 (70)	4 (10)	2 (5)
Money budgeting	3 (7.5)	18 (45)	18 (45)	1 (2.5)
Welfare benefits	20 (50)	4 (10)	1 (2.5)	15 (37.5)

Data from staff interviews (*n*=40) were used. CANDID, Camberwell Assessment of Need for Adults with Developmental and Intellectual Disabilities.

users and carers were significantly different, as were ratings by users and staff, (*P*<0.01). Table 2 shows the staff ratings for the 25 areas of the CANDID. The mean duration of the interviews at T_1 was 28.25 minutes (s.d.=7.84) for users, 29.56 (s.d.=6.52) for carers and 27.42 (s.d.=5.00) for staff.

Validity

Face validity

A number of different perspectives were taken into account during the development process, and comments were incorporated into the final version. Professionals from a variety of disciplines expressed the view that the CANDID is a comprehensive instrument covering a wide range of needs of people with learning disabilities and mental health problems. The CANDID, therefore, has acceptable face validity.

Content validity

All 45 users and carers approached responded to the questionnaire. Following the survey a total score for each need item was calculated and all items were ranked according to this score. The highest scoring items were accommodation and self-care, while the lowest were autistic features and telephone use. No additional items were suggested by more than two respondents.

Consensual validity

Forty-five experts (81.8%) responded to the questionnaire. Regarding the instrument's content, no item was rated as redundant and only 'communication' was suggested for inclusion by more than two respondents. Only 5% of respondents rated the instrument's structure as low for 'helpfulness of anchor points' and 'ease of use.' The draft instrument's language was rated as 'inappropriate' by 20% of respondents, and their comments were taken into account

in developing the final version. Thus, satisfactory consensus on the content and structure of the instrument was ensured.

Criterion validity

The CANDID summary scores (total number of needs) were compared with the total DAS and GAF scores. In both DAS and GAF, higher scores indicate higher levels of functioning, whereas high CANDID scores indicate high need. The Spearman's r correlation coefficients were −33 (*P*<0.05) and −47 (*P*<0.01) respectively, implying high concurrent validity.

In the individual areas examined (behaviour, communication, mobility, social interaction and self-care), the DAS scores were consistently lower for those assessed by the CANDID as having a need than for those assessed as not having a need, indicating an association between the DAS and CANDID in the expected direction. In the first three areas the differences were statistically significant and the respective mean difference values were 2.95 ($P<0.001$, 95% CI 1.63–4.27), 0.79 ($P<0.05$, 95% CI 0.60–1.51) and 1.2 ($P<0.001$, 95% CI 0.78–1.62). In the remaining two areas, where statistical significance was not reached the DAS items inquired about much narrower areas of functioning than the corresponding CANDID items.

Reliability

Intraclass correlations between summary scores of the two raters (for interrater reliability) and at the two points in time T_1 and T_2 (for test–retest reliability) were calculated using variance components analysis as described above. For interrater reliability the intraclass coefficients were 0.93 for user, 0.90 for carer and 0.97 for staff ratings. For test–retest reliability they were 0.71, 0.69 and 0.86 respectively. On the basis of paired t-tests there was no evidence of relative bias between the two time points or between live and taped interviews. In addition to total number of needs (section 1), the interrater and test–retest reliability of the summary scores for Sections 2, 3 and 4a were calculated. There was a high degree of agreement between raters and across time, and the correlations were generally higher for interrater than for test–retest reliability. The results are shown in Table 3.

Interrater and test–retest reliability were also examined for each need area item separately and two measures of agreement were calculated: percentage of complete agreement and k coefficients. Values of k in the range 0.81–1.00 indicate 'almost perfect' agreement with 0.61–0.80 indicating 'substantial', 0.41–0.60 'moderate' and 0.00–0.40 indicating 'poor' agreement (Landis & Koch, 1977). Only three k values were in the 'poor' agreement range; all were derived from user ratings and concerned test–retest reliability in the scores of self-care, information and welfare benefits. Values of the k in some instances were very low despite high complete agreement. Examination of the raw data in such instances showed that this was due to highly skewed distribution of scores. This difficulty with misleading k values is discussed by Feinstein & Cicchetti (1990).

For interrater reliability the lowest percentages of complete agreement on ratings of presence of need in a defined area were 71.0% for users, 85.1% for carers and 77.5% for staff; only 0.7% of the percentages were below 75%. For test–retest reliability the lowest percentages were 58.3%

for users, 66.6% carers and 71.0% for staff; only 4.7% of the percentages were below 75%. Table 4 shows the k coefficients for each need area item for interrater and test–retest reliability.

DISCUSSION

The measurement of need

Two conceptual issues underlie the difficulty in measuring need and are particularly relevant in people with learning disabilities. First, there is no consensus about the definition of need. The following definitions, among others, have been proposed "the requirement of individuals to enable them to achieve acceptable quality of life" (Department of Health Social Services Inspectorate, 1991), and "a problem which can benefit from an existing intervention" (Stevens & Gabbay, 1991). People with learning disabilities often have a complex constellation of difficulties commonly referred to as 'special needs', but it has not been established whether either the 'quality of life' or 'ability to benefit' approach (or indeed any other) contains the necessary and sufficient information for defining need in this population.

Second, there is a lack of consensus about who should assess need. Some argue that need can only be assessed by professionals (Mooney, 1986), whereas others (Bradshaw, 1972) claim that individuals' assessment of their own ('felt' and 'expressed') needs is valid. The combination of cognitive impairment, mental state abnormalities and behavioural disorders exhibited by adults with learning disabilities

and mental health problems may significantly affect their mental capacity. However, it is important to take into account the views of the service users themselves, especially if they differ systematically from those of other assessors (Slade, 1994).

Validity

A balance had to be struck between the utility and the comprehensiveness of the new instrument. The decision to retain or add items was taken on the basis of the balanced views of those who participated in the validity study. Accordingly, one item (communication) was added, whereas four (intimate relationships, autistic features, telephone use and medication) were not retained from the original list of items.

The lack of a 'gold standard' instrument necessitated the use of instruments that only indirectly measure level of need. Furthermore, it was only possible to compare five out of the 12 DAS items with the corresponding areas in the CANDID. The remaining seven either did not correspond to any CANDID areas or had their scoring based on different criteria, thus not allowing meaningful comparison.

Reliability

A difficulty associated with testing the interrater reliability of instruments administered via a semi-structured interview is that the second rater may be influenced by the interviewer. The rating of Sections 2–4 is dependent on the rating of the presence of a need in Section 1. Moreover, this process reduces the sample sizes available for

Table 3 Test–retest and interrater reliability for the CANDID

CANDID Section	Type of reliability	Intraclass correlation coefficient		
		User ratings	Carer ratings	Staff ratings
1 (total number of needs)	Test–retest	0.71	0.69	0.86
	Interrater	0.93	0.90	0.97
2 (help given by relatives/friends)	Test–retest	0.93	0.95	0.96
	Interrater	0.96	0.91	0.96
3a (help given by services)	Test–retest	0.75	0.90	0.88
	Interrater	0.98	0.96	0.92
3b (help needed by services)	Test–retest	0.72	0.87	0.84
	Interrater	0.94	0.93	0.94
4a (right kind of help?)	Test–retest	0.65	0.76	0.64
	Interrater	0.84	0.86	0.88

Reliability for sections 2–4 was only calculated for cases where there was an agreement between interviewer and rater on a need being present (section 1). CANDID, Camberwell Assessment of Need for Adults with Developmental and Intellectual Disabilities.

Table 4 Identification of need in the 25 areas of the CANDID: k coefficients for interrater and test–retest reliability

	User		Carer		Staff	
	Interrater (n=31)	Test–retest (n=24)	Interrater (n=27)	Test–retest (n=21)	Interrater (n=40)	Test–retest (n=31)
Accommodation	–¹	–¹	–¹	–¹	0.84	0.84
Food	0.77	0.78	0.79	1	0.33	–¹
Looking after the home	0.74	0.50	1	–¹	1	0.63
Self-care	0.87	0.29	1	1	1	0.48
Daytime activities	0.76	–¹	0.80	0.78	0.77	0.44
General physical health	0.91	0.88	0.91	0.80	1	0.81
Eyesight and hearing	0.87	0.73	0.93	0.91	0.95	0.92
Mobility	0.96	0.78	0.91	0.77	1	1
Seizures	1	0.88	1	1	1	0.91
Major mental health problems	0.94	0.54	0.86	0.64	0.87	0.61
Minor mental health problems	0.77	0.46	0.75	0.47	0.82	0.70
Information	0.75	0.40	1	0.50	1	0.68
Safety to self	0.70	0.47	0.93	1	0.96	0.88
Exploitation risk	0.89	0.73	0.73	0.46	1	0.71
Safety to others	0.80	0.64	0.86	0.82	0.92	0.75
Inappropriate behaviour	0.96	0.68	0.93	0.48	1	0.62
Substance misuse	0.96	0.46	1	0.50	0.82	1
Communication	0.94	0.69	0.87	0.66	0.95	0.65
Social relations	0.89	0.48	0.85	0.76	0.90	0.93
Sexual expression	1	–¹	0.86	0.53	0.81	0.82
Caring for someone else	1	0.66	1	1	1	1
Basic education	0.77	0.77	0.81	0.70	0.60	0.47
Transport	0.70	0.52	0.72	1	0.90	0.86
Money budgeting	0.58	0.62	0.72	0.53	0.83	0.53
Welfare benefits	0.90	0.29	0.78	0.79	0.92	0.84

1. k coefficients were not calculated because of one variable being a constant, marginal distribution being highly skewed or size being too small. CANDID, Camberwell Assessment of Need for Adults with Developmental and Intellectual Disabilities.

analysis and caution therefore is required in interpreting the reliability of Sections 2–4.

Generalisability

The reliability study sample was non-random and our research was conducted in only two sites, whereas there are large variations in the philosophy, structure and aims of services providing care for adults with learning disabilities and mental health problems in the UK. Nevertheless, an effort was made to make the sample as representative as possible by including service users from a variety of settings and with a range of levels of learning disability and associated mental or behavioural disorders.

Assessing needs from multiple perspectives is one of the main characteristics of the CANDID. However, the views of the service users are skewed towards the high end of ability, as individuals with severe and profound disability were not able to

rate their own needs. Although not investigated in this study, one approach for future work will be to assess the views of an advocate whenever it is not possible to obtain the views of the service user.

Implications for health and social services

A valid and reliable needs-assessment instrument for people with learning disabilities and mental health problems will be a useful clinical and research tool. The increasing costs of health care and lack of consensus about the most effective way of organising and providing health and social care have led government policy to be increasingly informed by evidence-based practice. The CANDID will enable rational use and fair distribution of scarce resources by encouraging needs-led service provision. However, the CANDID was not designed as an outcome measure, so other appropriate

instruments should be used when measurement of change over time is required.

The CANDID will facilitate the fulfilment of the local authorities' statutory obligation for needs assessment. It can be used for planning services, both at an individual level (developing individualised care plans) and at a population level (designing a service in a geographical area). The CANDID can, through systematic inquiry, help to identify areas of need that may require further exploration. However, it is a screening instrument rather than a diagnostic one and as such it is not a substitute for health or social care interventions, such as regular health checks.

As with the CAN, the need for separate versions for research and clinical use emerged during the developmental process. The findings reported here were obtained using the research version of the CANDID.

Two areas of concern about the draft clinical version have arisen: difficulty with its use in busy routine clinical settings, and the potential loss of useful clinical information caused by the structured nature of responses. The clinical version of the CANDID has adopted a combined approach: it uses the structured format of Section 1 to rate systematically the presence or absence of need, followed by semi-structured sections which allow the recording of relevant clinical information as part of the individual's care plan.

The findings of this study suggest that the CANDID has acceptable validity and reliability when used under the research conditions of this study. More data on its utility and feasibility are required; these characteristics will be established with its application in routine settings in the long term. A pilot study by the core research team aimed at investigating the feasibility of the instrument's use in routine community-based and in-patient settings is currently under way.

ACKNOWLEDGEMENTS

We thank all service users who participated in the study, their informal carers and keyworkers, and all the professionals who provided valuable comments on the various CANDID drafts. We thank Dr Rosalind Bates and all the members of the learning disabilities team at Bassett's Centre, as well as Dr Lachlan Campbell and the Mental Impairment Evaluation and Treatment Service team for providing access to the community and hospital services respectively. Special thanks to M. Phelan for his advice and support. We acknowledge the generous financial support of the National Health Service Executive SouthThames (R&D) by way of a research training fellowship (health services research) awarded to K.X.

REFERENCES

American Psychiatric Association (1994) *Diagnostic and Statistical Manual of Mental Disorders* (4th edn) (DSM–IV). Washington, DC: APA.

Audit Commission (1992) *Community Care: Managing the Cascade of Care.* London: HMSO.

Bradshaw, J. (1972) A taxonomy of social need. In *Problems and Progress in Medical Care: Essays on Current Research* (ed. G. McLachlan). Oxford: Oxford University Press.

Department of Health Social Services Inspectorate (1991) *Care Management and Assessment: Summary of Practice Guidance.* London: HMSO.

Dunn, G. (1992) Design and analysis of reliability studies. *Statistical Methods in Medical Research*, **I**, 123–157.

Feinstein, A. R. & Cicchetti, D. V. (1990) High agreement but low kappa: I. The problems of two paradoxes. *Journal of Clinical Epidemiology*, **43**, 543–549.

Holmes, N., Shah, A. & Wing, L. (1982) The Disability Assessment Schedule: a brief screening device for use with the mentally retarded. *Psychological Medicine*, **12**, 879–890.

House of Commons (1990) *The National Health Service and Community Care Act.* London: HMSO.

Landis, J. R. & Koch, G. C. (1977) The measurement of observer agreement for categorical data. *Biometrics*, **33**, 159–174.

Mooney, G. (1986) Need, demand and the agency relationship. In *Economics, Medicine and Health Care* (ed. G. Mooney) (2nd edn). London: Harvester Wheatsheaf.

Phelan, M., Slade, M., Thornicroft, G., et al (1995) The Camberwell Assessment of Need: the validity and reliability of an instrument to assess the needs of people with severe mental illness. *British Journal of Psychiatry*, **167**, 589–595.

Reiss, S. (1994) Psychopathology in mental retardation. In *Mental Health in Mental Retardation* (ed. N. Bouras). Cambridge: Cambridge University Press.

Slade, M. (1994) Need assessment: Involvement of staff and users will help to meet needs. *British Journal of Psychiatry*, **165**, 293–296.

SPSS (1996) *SPSS for Windows: Base System User's Guide. Release 7.5.* Chicago, IL: SPSS Inc.

Stevens, A. & Gabbay, J. (1991) Needs assessment needs assessment. *Health Trends*, **23**, 20–23.

CLINICAL IMPLICATIONS

■ The use of a valid, reliable and brief needs-assessment instrument for adults with learning disabilities and mental health problems encourages comprehensive needs-led individual care planning.

■ The Camberwell Assessment of Need for Adults with Developmental and Intellectual Disabilities (CANDID) allows the systematic collection of needs-based data which, when aggregated, can inform resource allocation and service planning in health and social care for this group.

■ The perspectives of service users and informal carers, as well as professional staff, can be assessed separately and taken into consideration.

LIMITATIONS

■ The sample for the reliability study was relatively small and selected from only two sites.

■ The structure of the interview meant that interrater reliability could not take into account the judgements of the non-interviewing rater if the latter identified the presence of a need when the interviewer did not.

■ Because of the lack of any relevant 'gold standard' for measuring needs in this group, concurrent validity was investigated using instruments that only indirectly assess need.

KIRIAKOS XENITIDIS, MRCPsych, GRAHAM THORNICROFT, PhD, MORVEN LEESE, PhD, MIKE SLADE, PhD, Section of Community Psychiatry (PRiSM), Institute of Psychiatry, London; MARIA FOTIADOU, MRCPsych, Lewisham & Guy's NHS Trust, Ladywell Unit, Lewisham Hospital, London; HELEN PHILP, BSc, JANE SAYER, MSc, Maudsley Centre for Behavioural Disorders, the Bethlem Royal Hospital Beckenham, Kent; ELIZABETH HARRIS, DipSW, The Green, Frant, Tunbridge, Wells, Kent; DONNA McGEE, RMN, Ravensbourne Trust, Farnborough, Kent; DECLAN MURPHY, MRCPsych, Department of Psychological Medicine, Institute of Psychiatry, London

Correspondence: K. Xenitidis, Section of Community Psychiatry (PRiSM), Institute of Psychiatry, De Crespigny Park, London SE5 8AF

The CANDID is available from the Section of Community Psychiatry (PRiSM), Institute of Psychiatry, De Crespigny Park, London SE5 8AF

(First received 17 May 1999, final revision 13 August 1999, accepted 17 August 1999)